PREPARING FOR
RESIDENCY

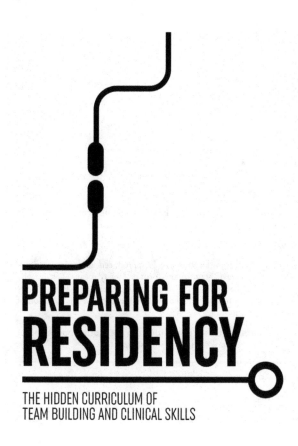

PREPARING FOR
RESIDENCY

THE HIDDEN CURRICULUM OF
TEAM BUILDING AND CLINICAL SKILLS

CHRISTOPHER LEE TAICHER, M.D.

For information about this title or to order other books and/or electronic media, contact the publisher:

Stone Age Publishing
outofthestoneage@gmail.com

ISBNs:
978-1-7354227-0-1 (print)
978-1-7354227-1-8 (eBook)

Printed in the United States of America

Contents

PART 2
Clinical Competence
~ 99 ~

Introduction

Medical students are often underprepared for their intern year as a resident. Some argue that the poor preparation contributes to the spike in mortality rates and medication errors that is observed during the month of July, when new interns enter hospitals and begin residency. This 'July effect' has been covered by major news sources such as *Time* and *U.S. News World Report*.[1]

I first published suggestions on improving safety in teaching hospitals as it pertains to interns on *The Boston Globe's* online STAT News site. The suggestions included having medical students work more closely with seasoned physicians to practice placing medication orders and increasing involvement in hands-on procedure simulations.

To better prepare medical students to transition to becoming physicians, it is necessary to improve on more than teaching medical skills in medical school. Resident preparation needs to focus on the two most pivotal "non-medical" skills to be an effective physician: *professional relationship dynamics* (or team building) and *clinical competence.* With respect to *clinical competence,* I refer to the skills that are needed in addition to a strong medical knowledge-base to deliver excellent healthcare. Knowledge base alone is insufficient. How can a physician be effective and deliver excellent care, even with all the knowledge in the world, if they lack bedside manner and tact in delivering bad news?

While team building and clinical competence are classically learned through on-shift experiences as part of the "hidden curriculum," this material can be taught in a direct manner before interns arrive at the hospital with MDs slapped on their white coats.

There is no guarantee that making the hidden curriculum more literal, as this text sets out to do, will have an impact on the July effect. However, because trainees commonly speak up about a lack of teaching on these subjects, and physicians identify these subjects as integral to a successful career, directly teaching about the hidden curriculum has potential to improve resident-driven patient care.

Learning *professional relationship dynamics* is clearly perceived as critical to a successful medical career by physicians. The 2019 Medscape study, including data from *fifteen thousand* physicians, elucidates this fact.[2] The study showed that *respect* from "administrators, employers, colleagues, and staff" was the fourth most important factor for personal sense of accomplishment and well-being.[3] And the *most important* modifiable one. While there were three more frequently cited contributors to physicians' mental well-being than respect, they were outside an individual's practical control (bureaucratic tasks like paperwork, work hours, and electronic health record utilization).

Thus, the first half of this text is a guide on how to navigate professional relationships in training, using residency as the primary example. It includes:

+ how to support your co-residents (including identifying and aiding burnt-out residents),

+ how to optimize patient satisfaction through evidence-based behaviors,

+ delicately handling several forms of challenging patients (angry ones, nervous ones, malingerers, and others),

+ how to encourage and realign nursing staff using patient-oriented language,

+ and when and how to stand up to mistreatment by attendings and other staff.

The second half of the book focuses on how to develop *clinical competence*, specifically skills that will help you apply robust medical knowledge, but which themselves are largely "non-medical."

I cover strategies for the following:

+ bedside manner,

+ distinguishing patients who need immediate attention from those who can wait ("sick" versus "not sick"),

+ tips to pre-rounding, including efficient utilization of the electronic health record,

+ how to represent yourself on rounds with organization and confidence,

+ integration of departmental "flow" into your treatment plans,

+ handling death and dying (discussing goals of care questions, sharing prognoses with critically ill and employing end-of-life care strategies that maintain dignity and optimize comfort),

+ delivering bad news to family and supporting your team with debriefing,

+ how to assess patient decision-making capacity,

+ on-shift self-care strategies,

+ and fostering an innovative mindset.

Now, what makes me qualified to write about such issues?

Honestly, I don't profess to be an expert. I have, however, had the good fortune to learn from a number of personal struggles during my own residency. I also interviewed over a hundred residents and attendings to learn about common struggles and successes. I conducted an extensive literature review on these topics as well, so the advice offered in this book is drawn from a wide base of evidence.

My own struggles in my residency training began with switching specialties from neurology to emergency medicine. I left my matched program in neurology at Albert Einstein / Montefiore Medical Center to join the Harvard Affiliated Emergency Medicine Residency (HAEMR) at Massachusetts General Hospital and Brigham and Women's Hospital. Making this change, I unintentionally contributed to the violation that the program received from the National Residency Match Program (NRMP). Being the person that gets your program dinged doesn't help you as a resident, at the very least from an internal guilt perspective.

At HAEMR, I faced immense challenges, both personally and professionally. Mid-training, I was called to a meeting by the directors and asked to "improve in every area of practice," from clinical acumen to interpersonal skills. Apparently, multiple faculty members expressed concerns about my engagement in training. One attending told me directly, "No one trusts you." Very confidence-building.

One reason I struggled was that I had too many outside commitments to focus solely on my residency, including drumming in a funk band called Astrojanit and gigging regularly in and around Boston.

By the end of residency, I made the necessary adjustments and drastically improved the way faculty members perceived me. I received unsolicited letters from co-residents and nurses about my improved clinical competence. I also received, to my great surprise, praise from attendings as a stand-out resident. And, most importantly, I was sent letters from patients about the excellent care they received. I was later asked by one of our program directors to coach a struggling resident—the final spark that inspired me to write this book.

My hope is that this book will offer strategies to help you lead the kind of residency life where every day you exit the hospital with a feeling of immense accomplishment. But that you also feel mentally calm, leaving you prepared to take on endeavors outside training.

PART 1

Professional Relationship Dynamics

1

Professional Relationship Dynamics

If you believe that learning skills that build professional relationships is too contrived, that simply "being you" is the best strategy, I encourage you to briefly suspend judgement and give this text at least a short read.

Learning skills to improve your professional relationships refines your general etiquette. And if there is any question on the utility of etiquette, consider how Amy Vanderbilt explains its value: "When we have an audience with the Pope, visit the White House, salute the flag, we follow long-standing customs that require specific codes of

3

conduct. Observing customs helps us feel at ease in situations of an official nature, knowing what is expected and how to behave."[4] The benefit of learning etiquette to feel at ease in various social circumstances extends to the hospital setting.

Professional relationships in medicine hold specific mores and expected etiquette, and as such, it is worth building your confidence in this arena. This will allow you to handle them with ease and focus as much mental energy as possible on clinical judgement.

Mastery of professional relationships can even be a life-saving skill. Consider a patient who wants to leave against medical advice, despite being severely ill. Maybe they are septic and are at a high risk of death without IV antibiotics. If you have the personal skills to gain their trust and convince them to stay in the hospital for antibiotics, you will likely save their life.

Further, if you are interested in distinguishing yourself as a trainee, you will have to be adept at handling a multitude of challenging personality types, including both patients and providers. This includes helping patients navigate challenging medical decisions and supporting colleagues through complicated cases or emotional lows.

The "just be you" way of thinking also contradicts proven models on professional success. There are skills that need to be learned. Brian Tracey has described how to obtain professional success by rigorously enriching interpersonal skills through the study of human psychology, negotiation, and language mastery.[5]

Thus, master the skills laid out below as you would any other—an instrument, a sport, or a language. Even without mastery, I think you can take away something valuable for your growth as a clinician.

An important warning: Many professional relationships in medical training will be extremely challenging. Many colleagues may not treat you with respect (at first). They may even like you, but there is a part inside of themselves that won't let them be cordial and supportive. DON'T LET THIS GET YOU DOWN.

The way that some healthcare providers mistreat others is a systemic problem and won't be discussed beyond a few comments here.

Why do people behave this way in healthcare? My hypothesis is that they are both disappointed and responding to how they were treated. Their reality never lived up to the idea that being a physician would provide an overwhelming sense of approval, the gold bullion of social currency. Thus, they try to enforce a sense of superiority (however undue and illogical) over others around them.

If one goes into any field of practice, including medicine, for any reason other than because they enjoy the day-to-day work, they will be filled with deep disappointment. This unhappiness may obstruct them from ever achieving overall competence because they lack a deep internal drive and appreciation for the work itself. And as much as this is an analysis of the root cause of dissatisfaction with professional life and the mistreatment in the hospital hierarchical system, it should also serve as a sincere warning to check your own reasons for entering this field.

Try not to let your parents push you to become a physician in place of another profession that you are actually passionate about. Garner deep insights into why you are going into the field and what the long road ahead looks like. While the job of a physician can be immensely rewarding, in many ways, it is a thankless job with stressors that will make the most resilient individual feel hopeless.

So, *think deeply about this,* especially if you happen to be early in your training process, a medical or nursing student, or pre-med. Shadow doctors to get a deeper understanding of the daily routine. Talk to residents at all stages of training and attendings of different specialties who have worked different career lengths. Ask as many questions as necessary until you feel confident that your reason for pursuing this career is that you actually enjoy the daily work. If you feel certain that becoming a physician will lead you to genuine fulfillment, read on.

2

Major Recommendations

Aside from your own deep satisfaction at work, your team's appreciation and respect for you is tantamount to your success as a resident.

When you go home after a long shift, you want to enjoy the peace of mind of knowing that your team valued and respected your decisions.

The converse would be if you go home after a long day with a sense that your team is disappointed in your work or dislikes your practice or your personality. Simply, if you are not liked, no matter how much medical knowledge or procedural skill you have, you will not feel accomplished at the end of the shift, year, or residency.

So, learn to cultivate all forms of relationships during residency, as this will undoubtedly bolster your confidence and overall wellbeing. You will regularly interact with other residents, as well as nurses, attendings, clerks, security officers, environmental services (commonly "janitors"), technicians in all departments (especially radiology for the emergency people), consultants, and, yes, even patients. Cherish each of these relationships.

How do you cultivate work relationships in the hospital?

Follow the advice below, which covers the following points:

1. Begin with good intentions.

2. Make a positive first impression.

3. Adapt to the conventions of your clinical environment through introspection and behavior-pattern identification.

4. Become an effective communicator.

5. Express gratitude.

6. Learn details of colleagues' lives and families.

7. Lend a helping hand.

8. Stand up for yourself.

9. Don't throw anyone under the bus.

1) The most important pointer is **to behave in a way that conveys genuine intent (or purpose) to "do good."** This means to be helpful to patients and colleagues while learning to be the best possible physician. In other words, have a sense of commitment, connectedness, curiosity, and enthusiasm for every aspect of training, as these foster the best-possible

interpersonal relationships and strengthen your resilience throughout training.*[6]

In order to convey an interest in doing good, you have to begin with good intent, which starts with pursuing medical training for the "right" reasons. With few exceptions, the only "right" reason to pursue a career is that you are internally driven by the enjoyment of the work itself (not necessarily every single aspect of it, but overall you should enjoy it).

---

* For related readings please see the following important papers: Salles, A., Cohen, G. L., & Mueller, C. M. (2014). The relationship between grit and resident well-being. The American Journal of Surgery, 207(2), 251-254.

Zis, P., Anagnostopoulos, F., & Artemiadis, A. K. (2016). Residency training: Work engagement during neurology training. Neurology, 87(5), e45–e48.

Girard, D. E., & Hickam, D. H. (1991). Predictors of clinical performance among internal medicine residents. J Gen Intern Med, 6(2), 150–154.

Berger, L. (2019) Where does resiliency fit into the residency training experience: A framework for understanding the relationship between wellness, burnout, and resiliency during residency training. Can Med Educ J., 10(1): e20–e27.

Wortham, S. (2004). The interdependence of social identification and learning. American Educational Research Journal, 41(3), 715–750.

For some, this is easy. They love everything about the work a physician carries out day-to-day, including in residency training. Others may have to reinvigorate their passion for being a student by reminding themselves that they enjoy, above all, practicing medicine.

Certain ideals that may drive many to decide to become a doctor—such as that it offers social currency like family approval or a steady income—can lead to personal and professional tumult. If you don't enjoy the actual work, you will also likely become a dud of a doctor. The anti-dud is created by enjoying the work itself.

Another reason life will be very challenging in training if you don't have the appropriate intention, is that people, whether or not they have studied psychology, naturally spot bullshit. You will suffer as a result of their skepticism of you.[7] If you are someone who does not enjoy the work, it will show in the form of "cutting corners," and your supervisors will see with ease if you don't do thorough history-taking or exams, and if you're not thinking deeply about a differential or workup. Think about an attending who has extensive experience and has seen resident trainees come and go for many years. They will almost immediately recognize a resident who is not genuinely passionate about their career.

A moment that taught me how authenticity in training (and beyond) is critical: As a preface to my med school class beginning our first week of clinical rotations, one of our professors asked the class to raise their hands and tell the professor a hobby that they like to do. A friend of mine put up his hand and answered, "ice curling" (he actually was competitive in the sport). The professor then asked the student to remain silent until he finished explaining how the game works to the rest of the class. This professor gave many details of the game, including what the equipment was called, how many players there were, the scoring rules, and so on. After a three- or four-minute description, he asked the rest of the class to raise their hands if they believed whether he was an avid curler or not. Much of the class, who had probably never heard of the relatively unknown sport, believed that he was in fact an avid curling player. He then asked Bud, the med student, what he thought.

Bud laughed. "No, none of that was correct." The professor asked Bud how long it took him to recognize that he didn't know a thing about curling, and Bud responded, "A few seconds."

The lesson was that if you really know your trade or field, spotting bullshit is simple. The practical application to clinical rotations, which I thought was quite elegant, is that attendings (and senior residents) know what is going on with you and your patients as a trainee. So be genuine.

Show up with the intention to be committed, connected to the team, curious, and eager. Maintain this internal position, and your outward demeanor will naturally convey that you are there to bring your best self to every lecture and shift.

2) **Make impressive first impressions.** This starts with being on time. Ideally, be early, which is one relatively easy way to gain respect by showing you value your team's time. Be consistent in this. Similarly, demonstrate that you value

your position by arriving groomed, well-fed, and rested.

Speak with confidence and candor. It always pays to express that you are honored to be joining a team and give some details about your background and achievements. Consider preparing a few short versions of your bio, so that if you are asked to introduce yourself in a group, you know what to say, briefly and professionally. By practicing a snippet of your biography, you're honing your workplace etiquette and alleviating potential social stress of having to create one on the fly. Just be careful not to be verbose with your achievements while offering some insight into what makes you unique.

3) Adapt to the conventions of your clinical environment through introspection and behavior-pattern identification. For example, if you notice (as I eventually did) that you are someone who tends to dislike suggestions from non-MDs out of ego or some misplaced self-pride, then you must adapt and remain receptive, especially in an environment that praises open communication. Otherwise, you will be seen as dismissive.

As I will elaborate in further detail in the Nursing section below, you have to trust the nurses, because they are likely more clinically capable than you are as an intern, and they can always add valuable input throughout your career.

I'll never forget when I was called to a patient's room at MGH for "respiratory distress" to find them with a traech, hooked up to the ventilator while they desaturated to 80% oxygen. The nurse threw me the bag-valve-mask and asked, "Are you gonna bag him!?"

I immediately thought, *Holy shit, how do you do that!? How do you hook a bag up to a traech!?* I (and the patient) was saved by my senior resident. But the fact that the nurse identified the first necessary step shows how capable they are.

The point is that regardless of the range of mal-adaptive behaviors that you may have, it is critical to be vigilant about identifying these behaviors so that you can change them. If you are perceived as someone who is resistant to adaptation, your team will have trouble working with you, especially if they view you as stubborn.

Consider the possibility that you are someone who tends to ask a lot of questions with little mental filter. You may tend to ask basic questions more readily than your co-residents. You then enter a clinical environment where a high level of know-how and confidence is praised. Maybe you are on a surgical rotation.

In this environment, if you are too frequently asking for help in order to seem like you are trying to learn, or that you are a team player, it may backfire. You could be perceived as someone who does not represent the team the way that is expected.

Rather, carefully observe your team's culture and adjust accordingly. In the case of this hypothetical surgical rotation, you may want to be deliberate and choose no more than one or two questions on rounds.

One last example comes from a close friend and resident who transferred from internal medicine to emergency medicine. This resident—let's call him Dr. Abe—thought that he was savvy and efficient by bringing his laptop into every emergency room to take notes on patients. The problem was that this created the perception that he was *inefficient*—and he probably was in an emergency setting. I am going to avoid a lengthy argument as to why carrying a laptop is inefficient, but suffice it to say that in the emergency department, in a large percentage of cases, you need two free hands. This resident was repeatedly told by attendings, senior residents, and me to stop using the computer, at the very least, because it reduced the team's confidence in him, especially among nurses, who coined him "the medicine resident." Even still, he continued to use the laptop for about six months, and it became a theme of negative feedback in his reviews.

Right or wrong, typing on the laptop impeded his success. Eventually, Dr. Abe acknowledged that his pattern of behavior was hindering his acceptance into the team, and he left that bulky thing at home.

The habits that have become cognitive crutches (like having a laptop to easily review medical history and labs) are difficult to identify in ourselves. But the more you look for them and become aware of them, the more likely you will be to pivot in a way that leads to success. If there are common themes in feedback, ignore them at your peril. Succeed with identification and modification.

As a bit of an aside, the likelihood that you will identify and correct maladaptive behaviors will be largely based on the degree to which you feel the need to do things in your own way. Doing things in your own way with your own style is, in fact, critical to maintaining your individuality. But you need to be aware that in some circumstances wanting to be unique can be harmful to your success as a resident, for reasons that vary from pure perception to actual inefficiency.

With respect to your team's perception of you, I offer this anecdote: I began my first few months in emergency residency always wearing a white coat. As a transfer from internal medicine, I was not only used to wearing one, it gave me a sense of pride to don it. However, residents in my emergency medicine (EM) program (and probably most other EM programs) rarely do so. The emergency team in my new program had a history of seeking out residents donning scrubs, not white coats, to help handle the highest acuity patients, because if a patient was coding or needed an emergent airway, the doctor in the white coat was thought of as a rotating resident without the necessary experience or procedural skills. Thus, while the white coat was largely a matter of optics, it held a practical meaning to the team. Once I stopped wearing one, nursing more regularly approached me for help with critical patients. This was helpful to my growth as a resident because I was exposed to and included in more patient treatment decisions, even if the supervising attending needed to be involved.

Finally, if your style of clothing, makeup, or otherwise ever comes up, simply ask yourself if your patients would gain or lose trust in you for your choices that give you a sense of individuality. Whether right or wrong, many patients would question excessive makeup or an unshaven beard, for example. Conversely, a tasteful approach to your appearance, including a well-groomed beard, is likely to be accepted. It may seem ridiculous, but we are in a service industry and have to take this into consideration.

4) **Become an effective communicator.** This is a skill that will serve you in the hierarchies of the medical edifice, patient encounters, and personal relationships.[8] Take time to read and watch videos on the subject, and practice applying what you learn. I understand that a book recommending other readings may seem annoying, but *communication* is too vast a subject to cover here, so I will offer a few invaluable resources.

Matt Abraham, out of Stanford, has produced incredibly helpful YouTube videos on communication, including "Think Fast Talk Smart."[9] He offers numerous communication strategies from using "Yes and . . ." phrasing as opposed to "But no . . . ," to developing a speaking format of "problem, then solution, than benefit." He also discusses techniques to gain control during challenging, even hostile communications. He suggests managing anxiety by being conscious of it and leading with questions. He also proposes ways to disarm someone in a charged emotional state with phrases like, "I can tell you're passionate about this issue." Labeling another person's emotional state is such a powerful communication tool that FBI hostage negotiators utilize it when speaking to terrorists and kidnappers.[10] Finally, Abraham shows how to buy time to think and how to answer difficult questions through paraphrasing.

Roger Fisher and William Ury's book *Getting to Yes* offers practical solutions to discord when negotiating, including how to separate **people** from the **problem**. Basically, try not to get emotionally entangled in your expression of discontent.[11] Recognize that deeply held values are going to vary widely among colleagues and that eagerness to understand another's perspective will lead to cooperation. Another solution offered by *Getting to Yes* is to focus on **interests** rather than **positions**. People take positions that usually stem from one of several personal interests (security, economic well-being, a sense of belonging, recognition, autonomy), and your ability to recognize them and address them appropriately is the fastest way to finding a solution to a conflict.

5) Express gratitude regularly. Medicine is largely a thankless enterprise, and you will go to great lengths for your patients. Sometimes you even revive them from death without so much as a thank you from the patient or their family. That's why when you go out of your way to acknowledge a colleague that did exceptional work, you are offering gratitude that might otherwise be absent.

Consider writing a letter acknowledging the outstanding work of nurses, co-residents, and other healthcare providers.

If you do, you will create allies. You build a strong alliance with the individual you are acknowledging as well as the administrators who recognize you as someone who takes the time to acknowledge effective members of the team.[12] The key is to find a balance of how often to communicate gratitude to your superiors. If you write a letter every week about someone doing something great, it probably dilutes the potency of your message.

6) **Learn details of colleagues' lives and families.** Ask questions, remember names, and keep up to date on their lives. This may be easy for some, and it may take a special effort for others, which is why I include it here.

While this task is mentally demanding in the middle of all that you are already learning during training, it will undoubtedly pay you returns. The only qualifier to this recommendation is to be aware of a more critical guideline, that when you are at work, focus on work, and be strategic about when you socialize.

7) **Lend a helping hand.** Do tasks that are not necessarily within your job description. Help nurses roll patients, take temperatures, "babysit" or monitor a psychiatry patient for a few minutes (if you have the time). When people see you going out of your way to make their lives easier, then, at a critical moment when you need support, they'll be there.

8) **Stand up for yourself against "wrong-doings" at strategic times with well-prepared statements.**

Medical training institutions are wrought with ego and hazing.[13] As a result, it is likely that you will be on the receiving end of hostile communication. The most important thing you can do is to go into training with a strong sense of what you will and will not tolerate.

If you tolerate too much inappropriate behavior, you will be teaching others that you accept mistreatment, and you will be targeted again. Everyone knows that there are some residents that no one bothers, and others who seem to attract disrespect.

Once you establish where you draw the line, the next step is to determine how you will deal with challenging situations.

Practicing different responses in your mind (or in front of a mirror) before they occur will prevent you from feeling stepped on because you will know how to respond when the situation arises.

This applies to when you have to stand up for your team (from co-residents to nurses). If you see someone being treated poorly, respond with your rehearsed dialogue. For example, when it comes to observing "intern hazing" beyond what you consider acceptable, step in and say something like, "She or he can be educated in a different way. Let's be supportive."

Saying something like this really is disarming. This also poses zero risks to you. Imagine a response from an attending: "None of your business!" They can't say such a thing. They will only feel embarrassed and gain respect for you as someone that stands up for others.

Of course, you have to pick your battles. Don't be the only person to intervene in every conversation. Strike a balance between speaking up without being outright argumentative. You have to practice standing up for your residents because undoubtedly you will see them being mistreated as underlings.

If you are unsure which unacceptable behaviors to act on, consider what I call the "Can I sleep at night?" rule. As it sounds, the rule says if you worry, you are going to lose sleep based on what you see, then *act*.

9) Don't throw anyone under the bus. Give criticism in private. Of, if you really have to in public, do so tactfully.

For example, if a co-resident forgets to throw away their sharps after a procedure, it's probably best to remind them by pulling them aside, not in the middle of rounds, humiliating them.

If you feel that a junior resident should have done something like order a CAT scan of the abdomen for a patient based on what you considered to be a concerning abdominal exam for a surgical process, don't yell, "I can't believe you didn't order a CAT scan!" Instead, consider asking questions politely and collegially like, "Are you worried about appendicitis?"

The opportunity to give others feedback will be rare early in training and will arise more often as you ascend. In senior years of residency, there will seem to be numerous opportunities to be critical of juniors, but use your criticism sparingly to avoid juniors viewing you as pedantic.

Hopefully, this has given a background, not taught in typical training curricula, on how to interact with your colleagues with integrity and the right touch. As a recap:

1. Begin with good intentions.

2. Make a positive first impression.

3. Adapt to the conventions of your clinical environment through introspection and behavior-pattern identification.

4. Become an effective communicator.

5. Express gratitude.

6. Learn details of colleagues' lives and families.

7. Lend a helping hand.

8. Stand up for yourself.

9. Don't throw anyone under the bus.

3

Co-Residents

Your co-residents can be among the most powerful connections you will make in your lifetime. They are also the team you will spend the most time with and the group with whom you will most often be compared.

The best way to strengthen relationships in training is to let your co-residents (or co-trainees of any provider type) know you have their backs. If they truly think you do, they can be incredibly strong allies who will advocate for you in many ways, from shift coverage to supporting you during professional and personal challenges.

Additionally, by tailoring your communication style to the idiosyncrasies of the individual trainee, you will improve the relationship dynamic and most effectively work as a team.

In summary, follow these essentials on optimizing team-building with co-residents:

1. Offer on-shift recognition and praise.

2. Provide positive feedback to leadership.

3. Offer regular check-ins, or support.

4. Identify and address burnout.

5. "Cover" shifts when needed.

6. Share information rather than being "the teacher."

7. Adapt your communication style to resident idiosyncrasies.

8. Place consults in a structured format.

9. Express interest in their academic and personal life.

1) On-shift make your co-residents look like superheroes. When they speak during rounds or lectures, listen for comments that you find valuable and verbally acknowledge them. Leave your own shyness in the dust, the best you can.

2) Alternatively, praise your co-residents in writing. You might send a brief email to a director or assistant program director recognizing a co-resident's hard work or clinical save, like if they made a challenging diagnosis in a nebulous case.

3) In addition to praising residents, offer support by checking in when they seem like they are having a tough day. But be aware that there is such a thing as too much support or support expressed in a poorly timed manner. This can have an unwanted demoralizing effect. For example, if you see a resident being mistreated by other staff and you ask your resident in front of a large group of peers who witness the event, "Are you okay?" you likely will not get as candid a response as if you take a more tactful approach and either offer support in private or phrase things differently. For instance:

"That situation probably would have bothered me, but I thought you handled it well. What do you think?"

Additionally, be mindful to avoid outright disingenuous statements absolving your co-residents if they need to improve a behavior or skill. False reassurance is not helpful to their long-term professional development.

BURNOUT

4) **The severity of burnout became apparent to me when a co-resident I knew checked himself into a psychiatry ward.** Had I known more about burnout, I might have been able to at least make an effort to help that individual. I regret not being

there for them and hope you can be there for your residents by understanding a bit about burnout.

Burnout is a syndrome brought on by workplace events that cause a combination of emotional exhaustion, unfulfillment, and depersonalization.[14] Residency offers the classic setup for burnout. It is as an incredibly stressful experience, especially with the number of hours required and the fact that residents are often far from home, lacking support systems from friends and family.

The data on burnout is astounding. In the previously mentioned 2019 Medscape study, including over fifteen thousand physicians, 44% reported being burned out, 11% reported feeling depressed, and 4% were diagnosed with depression. The equivalent of one doctor a day commits suicide in the United States, which is the highest suicide rate of any profession.[15]

Don't miss the opportunity to recognize burnout as I did, so that you can support your residents.

How to identify it is easy as long as you're looking: they are behaving exhausted (forgetful, sluggish, etc.), depressed, or are uncharacteristically disheveled. You might even see a resident in tears. Don't assume they have the support they need.

Find a way to offer your support. This is a bit trickier than identifying burnout because many residents will refuse help. Not only because they might be a private person, but other reasons as well, perhaps including that they don't want to appear vulnerable. I feel this latter reason is especially true in specialties where machismo permeates, like emergency medicine or surgical specialties.

When you do address burnout with a resident, the best advice I can give is to: (1) avoid condescending language, (2) reach out in a private manner, and (3) start with questions expressing an interest in offering support.

To do things privately, you may have to write an email or catch them at the end of a shift to see if they can step into a quiet room. If you are not already personally close with that colleague, consider it an enormous opportunity to build a friendship and really help someone in need. When you do offer support, you can ask questions like "How can I help?" or "Do you want to vent or talk about that case?"

If you feel that it is not your place to get involved, you can always consider pointing out your concerns to an attending or administrator. You aren't going to get the colleague in trouble as long as you are expressing concern for their well-being.

An important way to minimize your own burnout is to try to join programs that acknowledge it and have specific methods and systems in place to properly handle it. If you are already in your residency program reading this, this advice can apply when you search for your fellowship or first attending position.

However, if you are a medical student, consider asking students, trainees, and employees working at your potential program about burnout. Either via email or during your hospital visit, ask such questions as: "How many trainees left the program in the last year or two (attrition rate), and why did they leave?" "What are specific examples of existing resources for dealing with burnout?" "Are there counselors available? If so, what is their training, and what hours are they available?"

Don't worry about being seen as a complainer. You will actually sound competent and thoughtful as long as you are careful with your tone.

5) In addition to helping deal with burnout, have your co-residents' backs with a few specific coverage tactics. If they are running late, try covering for them without paging your seniors.

Offering to cover entire shifts if they need can also be a tremendous help to both of you. If you have a day off, and someone needs a shift covered, as long as you are rested, take the shift. This will go a long way if you ever need help. Everyone is in a different phase of life, facing unique struggles at different times, and it won't be long before you benefit from a resident covering you—either taking a shift from you for a vacation or switching lecture presentation dates.

Make sure you also focus on getting your co-residents off of their shifts on time. If you are coming on-shift, consider taking a task off their to-do list, like perform a procedure for them. Similarly, if you are overlapping shifts and notice they seem overwhelmed, consider taking on extra patients that day to ease their workload.

6) **When it comes to teaching a co-resident, your approach should be one of *sharing* information, *less* showing off what you know.** Try to avoid a pedantic, verbose, or holier-than-though style.

7) **Further, try and learn your co-residents' personalities, idiosyncrasies, and style of practice, and adapt your communication style accordingly.**

For example, in handoffs (or "sign-out"), when speaking to a nervous co-resident, expect them to ask numerous questions. Tailor a more detailed presentation for this resident and expect to spend five to ten minutes per patient.

More "easygoing" residents, or those with whom you've built trust, can get a brief sign-out, like this one: "sixty-year-old male with pneumonia, on room air, getting antibiotics, and admitted."

8) **When placing a consult with a co-resident you haven't met, have a specific format.** [If you know

the resident and have built rapport over time, you might be able to skip a specified format].

First, make sure to offer your full name and request theirs. Obtaining residents' names sets up accountability as a backdrop. It is also of practical value to know whom you have spoken to beyond "the orthopedics resident." If you have to reach them for immediate help, document your discussion in your note, or discuss the case with their attending, you won't have to track down who exactly you spoke to for the consult.

Additionally, make sure your consults, after introductions, *begin with your reason for consultation,* usually in the form of a question. Generally, avoid consults if you don't have a specific question or task you are asking for help with.

For example, if a patient has a peritoneal abdomen and you need a surgeon, it is better to call and say something like, "I'm calling to see if you think this patient will need ex lap [exploratory laparotomy]," as opposed to "this patient is in a ton of pain, and I don't know what's wrong with him." While your questions to consultants will become increasingly concise with experience, as long as you make an effort *to lead with* exactly why you are calling them, your resident consultants will appreciate you, and they will more readily formulate a plan to coordinate patient care.

If you don't lead with your question, the consultant will likely say something like "get to the point," or interrupt and ask, "why are you calling me?"

9) Finally, spend time learning your co-residents' interests, hobbies, and academic projects. This will dramatically strengthen relationships.

For example, when I learned that my co-resident was a Mormon, I tried to expand my cursory knowledge of the religion by reading up outside work. I was intrigued by the religion and would often bring up conversations on the subject to better my understanding of his culture. I think this process bonded us in a way.

During my readings on Mormonism, I also learned that in their culture, there is a proclivity for pre-prepared foods, and was then able to share a common interest: my love of the meal-in-a-bottle

Soylent drink that provided nourishment on many shifts.

Beyond your co-residents' cultures or religions, learn about their lives as much as possible, including their academic projects. Share a relevant paper that may offer more insight into their work. Even if they already know the paper, it shows you care. You can't learn everyone's research projects in-depth, but you can find out what they find interesting and read an abstract of a recent publication to discuss. Small gestures go a long way.

Finally, don't date residents unless you've spent a long time getting to know them first. There's nothing worse than uncomfortable interactions at work. There's also a narrow possibility that a vengeful partner could not only make work difficult but actively seek to get you in trouble. Please heed this warning. If you decide to ask a colleague or co-worker out, consider carefully and do so very rarely.

On that note, one of the most important pieces of advice one of my mentors, Dr. David Peak, gave me and my class on medical professionalism was this: "**It takes a lifetime to build a reputation, but only a moment to lose it.**"

Don't take this to mean you have to be perfect. Allow yourself the leeway of making mistakes without self-flagellation. The takeaway is just to know that if you do something of sufficient impact to damage your reputation, like dating too many people in your department, you will have trouble regaining it.

4

Patients

Patients should always be thought of as part of the healthcare team. To keep this vital member of the team content, it is clear from recent research that a major focus should be placed on *time-budgeting* tasks. According to a 2017 *Business Insider* study that included over a thousand patients, three of the top five factors that most improved patient satisfaction with their physicians were ease of scheduling, minimal wait times, and not feeling rushed.[16] The other two factors were knowledge of treatment costs and expertise of providers.

TOP 5 THINGS US PATIENTS SAY
IMPROVE SATISFACTION

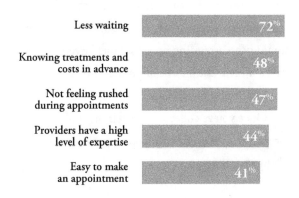

Less waiting	72%
Knowing treatments and costs in advance	48%
Not feeling rushed during appointments	47%
Providers have a high level of expertise	44%
Easy to make an appointment	41%

This evidence suggests that in order to impress patients, in broad strokes, you really only have to focus on a few simple time-budgeting tasks. Get to patients quickly, and then spend time carefully listening without interruption, showing them that you genuinely care.

Patients' focus is not only on their wait time until seeing you, but also how attentive and composed you appear, which can be especially challenging toward the end of your shift when you are more likely fatigued. Thus, stay vigilant about your performance at these late hours, and remember that patients do not really care about your previous patients, how medically complex they were, or how much mental and physical energy they took from you. A relevant analogy an attending once told me: "Every patient takes a little chunk out of you, and by the end of your shift you are a block of Swiss cheese."

Once you've collected yourself mentally and are prepared to engage with a new patient, do these things routinely:

1. Introduce yourself and make physical contact,

2. ask how the patient is doing generally, and if they are in pain,

3. focus on perspective gathering,

4. reinforce your interest during conversation,

5. convey your assessment and plan personably and

6. complete visits with an opportunity for patients to ask questions.

There are a few exceptions to this suggested routine on how you should carry out your exam, like caring for a patient who needs immediate resuscitation or if seeing patients while COVID-19 related precautions are still in effect, as it pertains to making physical contact (and if so, see below). But for all practical purposes, this should be your framework.

1) Introduce yourself and make physical contact when appropriate. Immediately get a sense of who is in the room, and start introductions with the patient. Shake a patient's hand or consider placing a hand on a shoulder. Some form of physical contact can be a therapeutic and relationship-building action. Most importantly, read the patient and decide what is appropriate. In the circumstance that COVID-19 precautions are still in effect, it is probably best to avoid contact unless donning the appropriate garb, including gloves, and you sense the patient will be comforted by it. Finally, when you deem it appropriate, shake the hands of a patient's friend or family member.

2) Ask how the patient is doing. (*How are you doing today? Or, What brought you in today?*) and then ask if they are in pain. When it comes to asking if a patient is in pain, note that by doing so, you immediately display compassion and interest in getting to the bottom of things. Just remember that if their pain is overt, like if they are writhing on their stretcher, don't insult them by asking whether they are in pain or for a pain-scale number. Tell them that you are sorry they are in pain and that you will order pain medication immediately.

3) Aim to understand the patient's perspective. As you delve further into a patient encounter, focus on understanding the patient's *perspective*. Think beyond history-gathering, and ask questions that broach the realm of how their disease has affected their lives as well as how their overall healthcare experience has been. To try and understand a patient's perspective on their illness is to create a humanistic foundation for your practice.[17] Specifically, ask a patient what their occupation is. If they are on disability, when was the last time they worked? What are their goals in terms of getting back to work? These questions need to be asked on a case-by-case basis, but they can get to the heart of their *perspective*.

4) Make good eye contact and don't rush. Part of conveying your interest in understanding how your patients are feeling is to sit at their bedside and make good eye contact. There is substantial evidence that sitting down at the bedside significantly improves perceived time spent with a physician, as well as bolstering rating scales on careful listening and communication.[18]

Eye contact is one way to convey that you are interested, and there are numerous others, like not interrupting a patient until they finish what they are saying, and then recapitulating what they've said. Some patients will be verbose or borderline tangential, and you can tactfully redirect, but try not to interrupt in the name of that important marker of patient satisfaction: patients *not feeling rushed*.

Preventing a patient from feeling rushed, as the data shows, is so important to a patient's perception of you that you need to have numerous strategies in addition to what was already mentioned.

If you find yourself feeling rushed because you are thinking of all the work you have to do, notes you have to write, or a procedure that you have to perform, ask yourself if it is really so urgent that you get to these tasks before cutting short on patient face-time?

If you are a senior resident with an advanced skillset that requires patients to answer only a few questions to arrive at your differential and treatment plan, consider asking what may seem like superfluous questions with the goal of increasing face-time with your patients. You may want to ask a few extra review-of-system questions or even where they are traveling from.

An additional strategy to augment face-time with a patient is to spend a little extra time in the room utilizing your computer to review the chart and place medication orders. Be mindful not to stare at the screen during your entire encounter.

5) Convey your plan in a personal way. When you are delivering your well-thought-out plan to patients, I believe it is best to imagine that the patient is a close friend or family member. When you imagine the patient is a cherished individual, you more easily relate to them, foster a rapport, and behave empathically when communicating your impression and plan.

Further, always be cautious not to talk down. If you've ever felt talked down to, then you know what this means. Another way to think about this is taking the stance of "sharing information and options," in place of "telling your patient what is going to happen."

Consider an elderly woman presenting with abdominal pain and dysuria, and your differential is UTI versus infected renal stone. Telling the patient your plan sounds like this: "You need a CAT scan, so I will go order it. I will let you know what it shows." Sharing information sounds more like this: "One of the concerns we have in emergency medicine with the kind of pain you are having is a kidney stone that can get stuck, become infected, and make you gravely ill. Instead of risking missing this diagnosis, I think the right decision is to order a CAT scan. Are you okay with this plan?"

On occasion, it is in the patient's best interest, based on their preference of physician style, to behave and speak in a more paternalistic style than in the "information-sharing" style.[19] A patient seeking a paternalistic physician wants to be left more in the dark rather than having you explain reasoning for imaging, for example.

You will quickly learn how to spot these patients. They may simply tell you their preference, or you may identify it in other ways. For instance, generally speaking, these patients consistently call you "doctor," are extraordinarily agreeable during the visit, and exude a "whatever you say goes" form of dialogue.

6) Complete the encounter with an opportunity for patients to ask questions. As you move to complete your patient encounter, always ask something along the lines of: "Is there any other concern or question that you have that I did not address?" or "Do you completely understand the plan?" These questions further clarify that you care that they feel as comfortable as possible in their healthcare journey.

Another reason you want to be thoroughly communicative is that it will help avoid litigation. The reason patients typically pursue legal avenues is that in addition to their original injury, the physician had poor handling and communication.*[20] If patients don't feel heard, they assume you don't listen or communicate effectively, and they worry you will propagate bad experiences and outcomes for future patients.*

---

* For more comprehensive characteristics of malpractice claims, please refer to the following:

Schaffer, A. C., Jena, A. B., Seabury, S. A., Singh, H., Chalasani, V., & Kachalia, A. (2017). Rates and characteristics of paid malpractice claims among US physicians by specialty, 1992-2014. *JAMA Intern Med, 177*(5), 710.;

Kornmehl, H., Singh, S., Adler, B. L., Wolf, A. E., Bochner, D. A., & Armstrong, A. W. (2018). Characteristics of medical liability claims against dermatologists from 1991 through 2015. *JAMA Dermatol, 154*(2), 160.

ESPECIALLY CHALLENGING PATIENTS

Now, we will discuss how to handle the most challenging types of patients: Those who are either angry (or rude, histrionic, or demanding), extremely anxious, malingerers, or neuropsychiatric patients.

The reason you should care to prepare for these patients is not only to make your life easier, but also for the unique opportunity to help others who are marginalized by the healthcare system, either due to their personality, lack of coping strategies, complex organic disease processes, or some combination of these factors.[21] Healthcare providers will often label these patients and be dismissive of them, but you have an opportunity to show them that you are different. Give the patient the pleasant surprise of fully acknowledging their suffering. When a nurse gives you a heads-up about a "difficult patient" in room two, eagerly accept the challenge, remember the lessons set forth here, and reap the rewards of having tactfully handled a patient that few have.

The more you understand why patients behave "badly" toward their healthcare providers, the more patience you will have with them. You will feel at ease handling them, and you will be eager to show your team your skills in this arena.

The causes of patient misbehavior are myriad. One interesting cause for the behavior is what I call *kindred confusion*. Consider a teenage male with a cold who curses at his mother while she brings him chicken noodle soup. Or a young woman in a hospital bed who tells her mother to "shut up" when the mother tries to add what she believes is helpful medical history.

These are examples of adolescents releasing their frustration on their mothers because they know their mothers will take the abuse without a dramatic impact on the relationship. Similarly, patients know that a physician has to (or at least hypothetically should) help them no matter how they behave. When a patient behaves rudely toward a healthcare provider, it stems from a sense of being cared for by someone that is supposed to unconditionally care for them. Basically, patients are confusing you with their parents.

Despite the reasoning for a patient's misbehavior, there are still boundaries, which we sometimes need to set. For instance, you should tell patients who are cursing at the staff, "You can't talk to our staff like that." But also remind the patient that you understand they are having a very difficult day, and that you are going to take excellent care of them.

As the first piece of advice when dealing with any difficult patient, whether while setting boundaries or otherwise, be mindful of your emotions. It is critical not to let yourself react to a patient's emotional rollercoaster. If you sense your heart rate rising, your muscles tensing, or that you are feeling antsy, take a breath and recognize that the patient is fueling your emotions, which is not usually conducive to a physician-patient relationship.

By recognizing your internal state, you can curtail maladaptive responses that are short or angry sounding, and instead stay composed and elevate your personal and caregiving skills through kind, tempered, and thoughtful communication. You will find that you disarm patients and change their attitude from angry to sweet when they recognize you will not react to their emotionally charged behavior.

ANGRY PATIENTS

To disarm the angry patient—someone who is already pissed before you enter the room because of how long they've waited or how a nurse "mistreated" them—apologize as soon as you introduce yourself. Apologize as an individual *and* on behalf of your team. Even if you are not actually responsible, the mere act of trying to take ownership of the problem will likely improve the angry patient's attitude.[22]

An apology acts as what the Goodenough Corporation, a group of American Psychotherapy Association board-certified counselors out of Seattle, calls "constructive confrontation."[23] I love this term because it describes not shying away from the patient and approaching them head on—albeit in a very kind and productive manner.

For example, if you tell a patient, "I wanted to apologize and take complete responsibility for the failure in our workflow today and how long it took me to get to you," you are more likely to appease a patient's frustration than if you said, "the hospital is really backed up right now." You can add to any apology, "Again, I'm very sorry that this is happening, let's focus on how to get you better." Shifting focus to getting to the diagnosis and treatment will also foster a happier patient.

HYPER-ANXIOUS PATIENTS

With patients who have anxious neuroses, they may have myriad questions, including what each review of systems question means and if their established specialists will approve all of your decisions. In these cases, the same aforementioned lessons apply; be mindful of emotions and apologize as needed. I also recommend that you behave in a reassuring manner through **formality** and **comprehensiveness**.

In terms of *formality*, I mean always introduce yourself to the patient with your full name and title, and also introduce each individual team member, especially nurses. Introduce yourself to not only the patient, but to all individuals in the room. This is helpful because such courteous behavior sets the stage for you as a thoughtful and professional provider. Anxious individuals thrive on reassurance. Further, by acknowledging each family member and friend with an introduction, you might assuage their anxiety as well, which can otherwise unintentionally transfer to the patient.

With respect to *comprehensiveness*, I mean that you need to spend a little extra time with that patient, including chart review, examination, and explaining workup results.

Before you enter a patient's room, know their chart intimately, including who their established providers are, and, if relevant, pay special attention to events in their most recent hospitalization. This way, you can further reassure them with a preface to your interview that you are familiar with their medical background. You may even want to give their providers a call, but this should be done on a case-by-case basis, as some providers may be bothered if you have not performed an exam and workup before calling them.

During your examination, check a few systems that you might otherwise glean or avoid altogether. This will prepare you to respond to their concerns about how their elbow pain might be related to their central nervous system. For example, "Since your neurologic exam is entirely normal, I am reassured this is not the cause of your symptoms."

In delivering any information to these patients, particularly your assessment, plan, and results, lean toward providing a bit extra compared to what you might provide to another patient. Telling these patients something like this is helpful: "Your kidney, liver, and heart tests, in addition to your white and red blood cell counts, and all electrolytes are all very reassuring." This is valuable to a patient who is generally anxious about something being wrong with them. So just think to give a little extra information.

Finally, with anxious patients, your confidence when delivering information is as important as the content. As soon as you demonstrate a lack of confidence, either by speaking in uncertain terms about a plan or generally sounding like you doubt yourself, you can quickly lose their trust. Remember to exude a confident posture and tone (without seeming arrogant) and avoid hesitation or vagueness.

MALINGERERS

Malingerers, any patients who like the hospital a little too much, are especially challenging. The approach to potential malingerers, or those with any form of factitious disorders, should start with your own certainty that you are not confusing potentially serious symptoms with histrionics. To avoid missing organic problems in those who have a history of "feigning" symptoms, assume patients who present with a possible fabricated disorder have an organically based medical problem until proven otherwise. This applies even if this is their tenth presentation in a single week. The most experienced physicians all have a story of missing an important diagnosis secondary to anchoring on a history of diagnosis of factitious or related disorder.

When you first meet a patient who could possibly be inventing a disorder, assume their symptoms represent true pathology, and, at the same time, look for potential inconsistencies in their story and exam.

For example, when such a patient presents with abdominal pain, you might want to try one of various distracting techniques to learn whether they are actually in pain, or feigning. My favorite distraction technique is after completing your initial abdominal exam, do a second concealed one, where you might tell the patient you are going to "listen with your stethoscope to the stomach", but you are actually using the diaphragm of the stethoscope to push down to assess for severity of pain. In medical school and residency, it is sometimes taught that either kicking the bed (to shake the peritoneum) or distracting the patient with conversation while you push on their abdomen also works, but I am not convinced of their effectiveness.

Once you suspect a malingerer, and you have determined that no further medical intervention is necessary, have a plan for how discharge is going to go down.

Before you enter their room, as with anxious patients, be well-versed on their medical chart. Otherwise, you may get ripped apart for not knowing some detail.

Any additional preemptive tests that you can complete to support the fact that they can be discharged safely should be done before you go to say your discharge goodbyes. Consider, for example, asking nursing or auxiliary staff to help with a food or liquid by mouth trial or ambulation (walking) testing, before you discharge the patient. A gentle reminder to patients that you and your team have observed that they can keep food down or walk with stable gait will convey certainty in a safe discharge plan.

Part of your discharge plan should include a clear explanation for how the patient can follow up with their primary care doctor, or specialist. Call the relevant provider to arrange this before you explain to the patient that they are safe for home. It is always reassuring if you can say, "I spoke with your doctor, Dr. Roberts, and we have come up with a safe discharge and follow-up plan." If you can't reach a patient's provider, write an email or leave a message, and let the patient know you have done so.

During discharge, remind patients that you are glad they came to the hospital to make sure nothing was wrong with them. Some will still be obstinate about leaving the hospital. You should remind them you are not only confident about their safe discharge, but that you believe it is wise to avoid the real risk of contracting nosocomial infections if they stayed in the hospital. If needed, give specifics:

> "About one in thirty hospital patients has a healthcare-associated infection. It also just takes one unscreened, asymptomatic COVID-19-shedding visitor to the hospital to get you sick. Or one healthcare worker who pushes through the shift with "just a runny nose." I'm so glad we don't have to keep you here and expose you to this potential risk."

One notable malingerer I encountered was a woman who presented with vomiting, demanding that her gastrojejunostomy (GJ) tube be replaced. Throughout her stay, she perseverated and insisted on replacement of her GJ, even after a fluoro study and CAT scan showed adequate placement of the GJ at the distal duodenum. The consulting interventional radiology team, who placed her device initially, felt the imaging confirmed acceptable placement. All the reassurance the patient was given, including from the IR team, wasn't helping her feel comfortable with discharge.

I asked what she was most concerned about if she went home. She responded, "I know I will start vomiting again as soon as I am home."

Fortunately, I had previously asked the nurse to trial liquids through the GJ halfway through her emergency department course, and so we had objectively shown that she could tolerate food and liquid. Reminding her of this fact, plus the reassuring workup and the consultants' agreement with the plan, allowed her to eventually accept her discharge.

NEUROPSYCHIATRIC PATIENTS

This ever-changing umbrella term includes myriad diagnoses such as personality disorder, somatoform disorders, certain chronic pain syndromes, and psychogenic non-epileptic seizure. They may pose the most challenging cases. While this is an enormous topic, I will briefly offer a few general recommendations.

First, **set expectations early.** For example, if a chronic pain patient presents with acute pain on top of their typical chronic pain, be forthcoming that you are going to do your best to relieve their pain as soon as possible, but that you don't expect to get them pain-free.

As with neurotics and malingerers, **contact the patients' physicians who manage them longitudinally.** Do this very early in their presentation. This will facilitate your ability to gain the patient's trust by explaining that you are taking a collaborative and personalized approach to their care. It is also a way of planning for the outpatient follow-up plan.

As with angry patients, do not react to emotionally charged expressions. This is especially important with patients with certain personality disorders, as they are known for emotional intelligence, astutely picking up on any change in your tone or attitude. Thus, you should stay extra-composed and regularly perform internal checks of your own emotional state during these types of encounters.

CONCLUSION ON "DIFFICULT PATIENTS"

You may have the inclination to complain about any of the aforementioned challenging groups of patients. While there is a setting to vent about your work stressors, the workplace is absolutely not one of them. Avoid the not-uncommon situation where a provider does not realize a patient is able to hear them from around a corner or through a curtain.

Speaking ill about a patient can lead others to judge you poorly—not only patients but also other healthcare providers.[24] For these reasons, I highly encourage you to take a position of never speaking badly about patients, regardless of whether you think you are in a private location. If you adopt this philosophy, you will not have to worry about being overheard or misinterpreted.

Further, if you have an impulse to criticize a patient, try and remember that patients rely heavily on you. It might help you maintain a compassionate mindset.

In situations where another provider is attempting to commiserate with you regarding a perception that your patient is annoying or inappropriate, respond with something like, "You know, he is having a difficult day." Try to kindly convey both your understanding of the patient's frustration and your disinterest in talking badly about patients.

One final piece of advice on relationships with patients: dating—don't do it. I have heard stories of the olden days when doctors and staff competed for a patient's phone number. Those days have ended.

5

Nurses

One of my most frustrating experiences in early training was being told by an attending that despite my hard work, several nurses had complained about me. Specifically, they had said that my attitude was a problem. I expressed remorse and an eagerness to remedy the situation. I asked for specific suggestions on how to improve. The response I was given was to "kiss the nursing ring," emphasizing the authority that nurses hold in almost any hospital or clinic.

My attitude problem stemmed from a need to display that a nurse could not possibly know more than a doctor, and that they were beneath MDs on the medical totem pole. This ego-driven perspective happens to be one of the three most common causes ascribed to physician-nursing communication breakdown: *hierarchal inequalities.* The other two are *role confusion* and *lack of trust.*[25]

If I had not made the adjustments to fully acknowledge nurses as *equal and essential* in the team, I would have not had enough nursing support to take care of patients efficiently, and I probably would not have graduated residency.

Nurses can and will take action to make life as a resident more difficult, especially if they don't like you. For instance, they could go over your head, straight to the attending, with patient updates or questions. Nursing might also bad-mouth you in ways that may or may not be accurate, but that will still tarnish your reputation. This can be detrimental, not least because you will be working with these nurses for many months to come (maybe years). If you're giving excuses, saying to yourself, *It's just this rotation,* trust me, it's not. Nurses from all departments talk to each other.

Given that nursing is integral to patient care as well as your success in residency,[26] please follow the advice below. Topics covered will be:

+ building nursing relationships by focusing on conveying respect

+ being conscientious of, and contributing to nursing duties;

+ delegating tactfully;

+ demonstrating confident leadership skills (including debriefing and protecting nurses' safety);

+ and knowing when and how to handle rocky encounters

To **convey respect**, *listen to nursing advice and integrate it into your plans.* This is essential for your relationship, but also for patient care, because nurses have tremendous foresight and experience, almost certainly beyond what you hold as an intern. When you become a senior or attending, you still must regularly listen to nursing. They have plenty to offer, and if you don't listen, they will feel undermined, which can cause them to resent you, seriously interfering with your training progression.

One way to let nurses know you value their opinion is by asking for it, even if you don't expect it to change your clinical decision. You might be surprised how much they can add to your assessment and plans in both major and nuanced ways.

I like to involve nursing in decision-making by asking, "I think Mrs. Smith would benefit from X, what do you think?"

You will have to find a balance of how frequently you ask for nursing input to avoid appearing overly reliant on others in general or, worse, incompetent.

Other ways to convey your respect include expressing gratitude toward the end of a shift by thanking nurses you worked with for their hard work and by writing acknowledgment letters to their superiors.

To be a **conscientious contributor** to the team, find a balance between doing some traditional nursing tasks, like placing an IV, and letting them carry out the work on their own. The residents who nurses consider to be the most willing to do tasks like boost a patient up in bed, place an IV, or simply get a blanket for a patient, are the ones who establish the most cred. This considerate behavior makes training easier and paints you as a team player.

Tactfully delegating tasks is immensely important. When it comes to delegating nursing work tasks, be cautious before interrupting nurses' work flow to make a request, so as not to undermine their choices and interfere with the patient care they are delivering at that moment. Unless you need to recruit their help for a critically ill patient, never interrupt a nurse mid-procedure, like when they are placing an IV or Foley catheter. This includes poking your head into a room to ask a question or submit a "basic" request like "the patient in room nine needs an IV!" This is rude and will piss nurses off.

When you do ask for nursing assistance, do not be intimidated. If you act as if you're afraid of nurses when asking for help, they won't trust your decisions. And you will also be less likely to ask for help when needed. Unfortunately, this fearful behavior is common and detracts from the confidence of the team as a whole, so be calm and direct instead.

Especially when it comes to true emergencies like running cardiac arrest resuscitations, nursing looks for one person to make confident, unidirectional decisions without seeking outside opinions.[27] You can still foster a collaborative team environment by punctuating your decisions with a request for the team's thoughts and concerns. However, a resident who knows when to step up and delegate is highly valued.

When asking a nurse for help, always consider *the complexity of the task* you are asking. Just like residents, nurses' experience and competence varies widely. And nurses, just like residents, are green and relatively inexperienced when they are new grads. The only difference is that nurses aren't as clearly distinguished by their years of practice as interns are (i.e., a new face, a short white coat, or scrub embroidery) so you may have to pay closer attention to understand different nurses' experience levels. You should also be aware that nursing tasks vary based on hospital rules and protocols. For example, in some hospitals, nurses, if trained, are allowed to place ultrasound-guided IVs.

Thus, be aware of not only a nurse's experience but also of the clinical environment when asking for help. If you are ever unsure whether a nurse can confidently carry out a task, you should ask them if they feel comfortable doing it.

Once you get to know your team of nurses well, you will know each nurse's skill sets, training background, and seniority (including time in the department), and you will spend less time confirming comfort levels with various work tasks.

Nurses may also feel uncomfortable stepping in late in a patient's hospital course, especially in delicate situations such as critically ill or end-of-life scenarios. Some may be concerned about liability around complex and dying patients. Just be aware that if you are going to ask them to get involved in these circumstances, you may need to take a little extra time communicating, including summarizing what has already happened with the patient and what the plan is moving forward.

A common instance that also requires you to spend extra time communicating (and sometimes taking other action), is when nurses or not cooperative. This may seem crazy (depending on what stage of training you are in), but you will eventually experience this: when a nurse needs more than a little encouragement to realign with the treatment plan, is behaving slothfully, or, in the more egregious situations, when they are intentionally making your life difficult. This unfortunately occurs at the expense of patient care.

Some nurses will be slow-moving to establish an IV on a hypotensive patient, or they might not reassess a patient by rechecking vitals when they should be. Whatever the lackluster behavior is, you will need to find ways to deal with it effectively, both for your sanity and for your patients' care. Any inclination to simply report all of these instances will be ineffective, and you will be viewed as a whiney character—not to say you shouldn't report egregious misbehavior.

The better approach is to follow these steps *(note: if the first one succeeds, you need not continue down the list.):*

1. Encourage the patient's nurse.

2. Do it yourself.

3. Implore another nurse.

4. Find the charge (boss) or "flow" nurse.

Let's start with the example of a nurse responding to one of your requests with something like, "I'm busy with another patient."

Gentle encouragement in the form of a question sometimes works. *Could you help with the new patient?* Don't be timid when you ask them to switch their task, as long as you find it necessary.

If you do feel timid, maybe it is because you are too timid in general, or perhaps you are inappropriately interrupting a nurse's patient care, which they should be prioritizing. As long as you approach these interactions with kindness, confidence, and consideration for the fact that nurses are caring for numerous patients, they will likely help you. Confidence is key because without it, nurses are uncertain if what you are asking really holds importance. If *you* aren't sure if they should switch tasks, why should *they* be?

Next, if a kind and confident request fails, encourage them by using language emphasizing **shared goals of patient care.** As already mentioned in the general recommendations section of this book, *Getting to Yes* contains a comprehensive list of ways to establish aligned goals within a team. As a brief reminder, use "we" instead of "I," and focus on what "the patient needs" instead of "what I need." *We really need your help with the patient in room four, their blood pressure is tanking.*

Another encouraging strategy is flattery. Tell a nurse you need their "expert hands" or "their IV skills in room four."

Note that timing is critical. You want to make requests for patient care when the nurses are the least flustered and not when they are already carrying out a task for another patient.

However considerate and strategic you may be, a nurse may still react negatively to a request to stop what they are doing and switch to a different task. This reaction can be rooted in a feeling that their ego is being attacked, as they are being told by a younger or less experienced person what they should be doing. Have compassion, and don't let their frustration affect your mental state.

In the off chance a nurse responds negatively to all of your requests, not taking helpful action, it is often better to abandon the encouraging approach and **do the task yourself**.

When you take it upon yourself to place an IV and draw labs, this is typically viewed in an extremely positive light. Don't do the task for its own sake, but if this is the best available option, you should take the initiative to keep workflow moving. It can be a great confidence builder in terms of your team's perception of you. If you think that you shouldn't know how to place IVs in your specialty, ask yourself: Do you really want to be a medical doctor who can't place an IV?

Asking nurses to do small tasks that you could easily do (or learn), like inserting an IV or taking a temporal temperature, can also get on people's nerves. I encourage you to learn how to do "the basics" of every process within your department so that you can take action when needed to maintain departmental flow. Trust that a nurse will be pleased when you ask them to teach you *(early on in your training)* how to most efficiently attach a modified oxygen saturation digital monitor or how to send tubes to the laboratory.

I make the side note of asking nurses to teach you *early* in training because this is when staff, in general, is most willing to help. As you become more senior, others will expect more from you. They will have less patience to teach you the fundamentals.

If you simply don't have the time or skill set to do a task the nurse should be doing, find another nurse. Just take care not to verbally degrade the primary nurse. Sometimes it is best to let the primary nurse know you are going to ask someone else to help because you understand they are busy. It seems laborious, but you can quickly give someone a heads-up and avoid making them feeling incapable or circumvented.

Similarly, don't speak ill of a nurse when requesting another nurse's help. Just say something like, "Kristin is really swamped right now; any chance you could help us out?" The last thing you want to do is complain about one nurse to another for the sake of your reputation.

Finally, if you've exhausted all options and still need a nurse to help with a critical patient, go straight to the charge nurse and let them know that the primary nurse is unavailable and that you need their help.

HUDDLES AND DEBRIEFS

An additional approach that will benefit your relationships with nurses is coordinating "huddles" and "debriefs" (or "decompressions") for challenging clinical scenarios.[28] These team conversations can occur before or after the scenario being discussed.

For example, if you get an EMS call or communication from another hospital's staff that your team is receiving a coding or critically ill patient, you can and should huddle with your team to create a game plan, so that the moment the patient arrives under your team's care, you act as a well-oiled machine. For instance, if an ambulance called in with a cardiac arrest, assign roles to providers (who is getting IV access, placing shock pads, drawing and giving medicines), get all team members to don protective gear and communicate to the team what you think are the likely culprits of the arrest based on the information you have.

These small staff huddles are also effective in coordinating a pre-emptive plan for speaking with those "difficult patients," especially prior to discharge.

Similarly, debriefs can be team conversations held after an event so that the team can learn from it. For example, if a patient dies despite resuscitation efforts, it can be crucial for the team to discuss the situation. Include all staff in these huddles, from nursing to the front-desk clerk who briefly

interacted with the patient's family, to the medical student standing in the back. Use the opportunity to obtain feedback from everyone on the team as to how you might improve your own clinical skills, tackle hospital systems issues, and address and support the staff's emotional and mental state. By creating an environment of inclusivity and open feedback, you show your leadership and provide a place for your team to connect; they will appreciate this immensely. A potentially obvious but important note is to hold these debriefs in a private location.

SAFETY

Protect nurses from aggressive patients and shield their risk of occupational exposure, like needle sticks. They will value your conscientious efforts to focus on their safety.

For patients who you deem a safety risk (either from reviewing their chart and noting past violent behavior or from observations you make), call for security bedside, or simply notify security to stay on alert. You may also want to remind a nurse of some protective strategies, such as not getting too close to a patient, or avoiding getting cornered in the room. Most nurses will have training on the subject and can intuit these strategies. Your reminders or suggestions simply convey your care for their safety and build trust.

Additionally, safety considerations can be difficult to remember if a chaotic code was just run. There may be sharps on the bed from IVs or a crash central line, so be sure to remind everyone to take caution until you can clear the bed. Also warn your team about blood and other biologic fluids that they could come into contact with.

ROCKY ENCOUNTERS

The final recommendations I offer on nursing relationships has to do with handling contentious interactions. The best general approach is to expect to be disrespected or questioned, because it will inevitably come up when you start training, whether you deserve it or not. **But let it roll off your shoulders.** Display that you aren't going to respond, either squeamishly or aggressively. This will empower you with the insight that you can handle the situation and it will make the disrespectful confrontations less likely to recur.

Next, make a mental note to find the right moment to pull a nurse aside to speak to them. You don't need to make the interaction a serious one. But acknowledge their behavior toward you. In these cases, the best way to start building a collegial relationship is to start with an apology. Apologize for nothing in particular if you aren't aware of what particularly offended them. But acknowledge you might have done something. Say something like, "I'm sorry for whatever I did to upset you. Sometimes I can be oblivious, but I want you to know I am sorry, and I would really like to work well together for our patients sake." The act of apologizing shows that you are open to critique, friendly, and approachable. The nurse will likely change their tone to one of forgiveness.

If you find an apology to be especially uncom-fortable, still try. If you are absolutely unable to, make a friendly gesture to convey your willingness to be collegial with that nurse. It might be as simple as bringing them a cup of coffee or a bagel.

Another potentially contentious situation to beware of is when a nurse is advocating for a patient plan of care that conflicts with what you deem to be the best clinical decision.

For example, a patient really wants to be discharged because they have been in the hospital "too many times," and the reason they are in the hospital to begin with is ostensibly bogus. The nurse says to you, "Her blood pressure is always low. Why are we admitting her?"

In these situations, do not get frustrated, do not take a nurse questioning your plan personally, but do consider that they may be right. But if you still disagree with them, use realigning language with the message that you are also advocating for the patient's safety. Provide clear and succinct reasoning as to why you are making your decision, which should ultimately hinge on patient safety.

Finally, as with co-residents, don't throw nurses "under the bus." For example, never reveal your disagreement with a nurse in front of a patient.

I once told a patient that the nurse had probably caused a bad reaction by flushing the medication (metoclopramide) too quickly. This undermined the therapeutic relationship between the nurse and patient. Remember that nurses spend the most time with your patients and they depend on you to support their decisions.

6

Attendings and Directors

Integrating the wisdom of providers you respect is what residency is all about. Identify attendings you admire, those who you believe practice with utmost excellence, and learn the reasoning behind their decisions.

Do this by asking **why** questions. "Why did you choose to admit as opposed to placing them in observation?" "Why did you choose broad spectrum antibiotics as opposed to just covering narrowly?" "Why did you choose to order a CAT scan of their chest instead of just stopping at a chest X-ray?"

One critical caveat: your questions should match your level of training, or what year you are in—try to avoid being "too basic" if you are a senior nearing graduation. This is because it can jeopardize your integrity with the team if the questions seem too basic given your level of training. If you are unsure whether the question is too simple, then it probably is. You can always look it up on your own or ask a co-resident to help you in relative privacy. I guess there *are* dumb (-sounding) questions after all. At least in residency.

In addition to finding your mentors and asking them **why** questions, for your success as a resident you need to gain the approval of **most** attendings in your program. This is how you guarantee graduating on time and working cohesively on-shift. My most important pointer to obtain overwhelming attending approval? Identify both the general practice styles and idiosyncrasies of each attending in order to adapt your practice to satisfy what they are looking for in a resident.

ADAPT TO ATTENDING PRACTICE STYLES

Below, I will lay out the categories of attendings' styles. I'll explain how to mold your practice into what they see as "the model resident."

Before that, though, I want to address a potential concern: *that it is unfair to be evaluated in an ostensibly subjective, variable manner by different attendings.* Medical practice varies tremendously from attending to attending, and so will the way they gauge your skills. This is because attendings, like all people, come from varied cultural and training backgrounds.

Also, don't forget that scientific literature is not so black and white. It can be interpreted in a variety of ways, and thus contributes to varied practice styles. Further, guidelines from scientific literature are ever-changing. Thus, you will grow to admire different attendings whose practices diverge from one another.

Thus, while it may seem unfair to be at the whim of an attending's gestalt opinion of you as a clinician, it is for now the only form of residency evaluation that exists, and you should accept it to avoid an unnecessarily frustrating training experience.

CONSERVATIVE ATTENDINGS

Now, onto attending types and how to handle them, starting with "conservative" attendings. *Conservative* is a relative term, but here we will use it to mean an attending who praises traditional, lengthier presentations (detailed exams and exhaustive differentials) and extra testing in general (like a broad array of bloodwork and imaging). These attendings tend to be more risk-averse. But they are actually easy to work with as long as you identify them. In these cases, simply match their behavior, **be thorough in your presentations, give a detailed history of the patient's present illness, lean towards providing a broader differential, and order a few extra studies to rule out highly unlikely, but concerning potential diagnoses.**

CHILL ATTENDINGS

On the other end of the spectrum is the "laid-back" attending. These individuals are generally perceived as being "chill" or "easy to work with," and they will generally provide above average evaluations across the board. You won't have to do much to gain their approval. The most challenging part about working with them is that residents often report a paucity of teaching from them. There's not much you can do to change this other than frequently asking about their specific areas of interest and requesting that they teach you.

EVERYTHING IN-BETWEEN ATTENDINGS

Finally, the "everything in between" style of attending (living somewhere between conservative and laid back) will require your flexibility. In these situations, ask directly what they are looking for (which still may not give you helpful feedback), and learn to read between the lines. Ask with genuine interest, "What exactly are you looking for in [presentations/exams/ differentials]?" If the answer feels insufficient, and you are unable to rearrange your approach, it may be that the attending has difficulty articulating their perspective or has not thoroughly considered what criteria they use for evaluation.

If you feel awkward asking directly or their answers are unclear, read between the lines. Here's how:

1. **Pay attention to attendings' interactions with other residents** (juniors and seniors), and notice what they praise and what they criticize. If you do this with careful observation and adapt your practice accordingly, you will quickly have their approval as a trainee.

2. **Watch for attending idiosyncrasies** during their patient history-taking, examinations, and lab and medication orders. If during exams, for example, an attending always checks gait stability, "walking his patients," start doing the same and "road-test" all of your patients. When the attending notices you walking down the hall with your patient as you support them, or that you are including gait stability in all of your presentations, they will appreciate your actions.

Likewise, if an attending gathers social histories on all their patients, including smoking and family cardiac disease, ask your patients for these historical components and add them to all of your presentations, even if you deem this information superfluous.

If certain patient chief complaints trigger a predictable constellation of lab and imaging tests or dispositions and plans, start parroting them when you are working with that attending. For example, if a specific attending orders an abdominal CAT scan on all elderly patients with abdominal pain, lower your threshold for including one in your workup. And when presenting your treatment plan, include an explanation of considerations you've made toward obtaining a CAT scan, such as ensuring the patient has a sufficiently large-gauge IV placed to administer contrast if imaging is needed.

SUPERVISOR MISBEHAVIOR

Supervisors are people too. Do you have a plan on how to handle it if your attending acts out of line, or misbehaves? You may see an attending rudely talk down to a young resident. "Are you kidding me, you don't know that!?" they might say. Worse, you may even experience a sexual advance from a boss while on shift.

I recommend first *staying calm.* The last thing you want is to have to defend yourself later for being inappropriate even when it was reactionary, or truly warranted.

Next, send the message that you (or whomever you are speaking on behalf of) are not going to be walked on. This is important because if you tolerate shit behavior, you are projecting what you will continue to allow.

You have to read the situation and the attending in each case, however. Consider reacting to an attending's belittling comments with anything from "Dude, that's not cool," to "That's not very professional. I'd appreciate it if you did not speak to me (or her or him) that way."

If belittling recurs even after you've addressed it, add "This is getting inappropriate," and "This is why we have the [society of such-and-such] to advocate for residents who are put in this situation."

Speak in a non-threatening tone, just state it as a matter of fact. This will likely put an end to the misbehavior because in medicine, people tend to fear any formal reprimand by a superior, especially an advocacy group.

If you find yourself receiving or observing inappropriate physical advances on-shift, you still need to first *stay calm, and get to a safe physical space.* Then, it is generally best to speak up. In these circumstances, be emphatic and stern to convey that you won't tolerate harassment. There are myriad ways to do this, including raising your voice or taking an austere tone to respond with: "You are completely out of line, and this will be reported." If you prefer to drive the message home more strongly by cursing, just be aware that you may be unfairly reprimanded for being inappropriate and compromise your position in making a formal complaint if staff overhears only the part of the conversation where you are insulting your supervisor. Nuances aside, **speak up when you see misbehavior,** whether it is directed at you or your co-residents. They will deeply appreciate you for it.*

One close friendship I still have today began after I defended a colleague from inappropriate hazing-type language coming from the attending cruelly criticizing her morning rounds presentation. I said something like, "We don't need to be like that when we teach each other, I am sure everyone will learn better if you kindly correct us. We've all been there early in training." Not only did this start a lasting friendship, rounds were a lot more comfortable and productive.

ATTENDING TO ATTENDING

Finally, a word on dynamics with other attendings once you become one: the hierarchy never

---

* For specific strategies on handling and prevention of gender based violence in hospital settings, please see:

Khubchandani, J., Kumar, R., & Bowman, S. L. (2019). Physicians and healthcare professionals in the era of #Metoo. *Journal of Family Medicine and Primary Care, 8*(3), 771–774. https://doi.org/10.4103/jfmpc.jfmpc_228_19

disappears. Some attendings in practice twenty years will still want to make sure you know you are more junior, and they will often question your management decisions. Maybe these senior attendings are genuinely interested in teaching, or maybe they feel threatened by a younger co-worker and need to display their seniority. Regardless of the reason, it can be helpful to respond graciously, and consider pointing out that you notice their attitude. You may say you don't appreciate their tone if it is hostile, but don't be defensive, as this can be divisive.

Further, to integrate yourself as a teammate and show that you value your senior attendings, share your cases with them and ask their advice, intermittently.

As discussed above, an important caveat to asking for your colleagues' advice is to *be cautious with the frequency you ask for it*. Ask for advice often enough that you are being inclusive, displaying open-mindedness, and eagerness to work as a team. But not so frequently that you may be viewed as too insecure to practice independently.

7

Auxiliary Staff

Relationships with auxiliary staff are the most underappreciated. This staff controls so many vital tasks related to your work efficiency. For example, when you need a room cleaned for a patient, a medical supply in order to perform a procedure, or any old favor, these are the people you count on. And when the staff who performs these tasks genuinely likes you, they will speedily and readily assist.

Thus, treat all auxiliary staff, from administrative assistants, clerks, and stewards, to volunteer, custodial, and security personnel, with as much gratitude and respect as possible. Regularly thank custodial personnel every time they clean your work area. Write a letter to their supervisor commenting on their positive attitude and initiative. Bring your clerks coffee or a potted flower. Spend some time asking security staff where they're from. People generally appreciate when someone unexpected asks about their life story.

Overall, as long as you go out of your way to thank, be helpful to, or get to know support staff, you will be repaid in spades. You will not only garner their respect and improve work efficiency, you will also feel proud of your job by including everyone and valuing all of the members of your team.

PART 2

Clinical Competence

The second half of this book explains how to succeed with techniques that optimize clinical competence. The first and most important technique, which may sound cliché, **is to enjoy the process of each learning opportunity.**

While the guidelines set forth below will also help you improve upon professional relationships, the recommendations that follow fit more within the domain of clinical competence.

8

Major Recommendations

1. Enjoy the process.

2. Accept failure.

3. Practice mindfulness.

4. Maintain composure.

5. Listen and provide feedback carefully during sign-out and team huddles.

6. Own your level of training.

7. Have humility during successes and saves.

8. Maintain a balanced civilian life, with a focus on hobbies and organization outside work.

9. Be as involved as possible in your program.

1. Enjoying the process will improve your mental well-being and it will improve patients' perception of you as a warm individual who is content to be in their presence. You shouldn't necessarily welcome suffering patients with a big smile and a spring in your step, but generally speaking, patients appreciate physicians who appear to like what they do.

Enjoying the process of training means you will also welcome learning opportunities, including seeing as many patients as possible and studying often and with a focused mindset. These actions lead you to retain more clinical information, expanding your knowledge base and critical thinking skills.

Follow the example of Jimi Hendrix. He was able to effectively practice eighteen hours a day *because he liked what he did,* turning him into a virtuoso that created works like the album, *Band of Gypsys.*[29] If you are able to find a way to make training into an enjoyable experience, you will stay open to more clinical experiences and you will mature clinically.

In contrast, a resident who does not enjoy the process will be reluctant to see more patients because they don't like adding work. Perhaps this person feels overwhelmed, that there is "too much to learn" or that "things are too hard." These attitudes prevent them from putting themselves into new learning situations, and thus limit their possibilities in terms of achieving optimal clinical competence. While residency will present you with plenty of opportunities to feel overwhelmed, resist despair and let your self-doubt be transient. Foster the mindset that constantly learning is enjoyable.

2. Accept failure. Acknowledge that residency will be a challenging experience with repetitive trial-and-error. **Foster resilience in the face of mistakes and missteps.**

Dr. Sam Collins, a social entrepreneur and motivational speaker named by Her Majesty the Queen of England as one of the Top 200 Women to Impact Business and Industry, put it this way: "Someone who survives failure has gained irreplaceable knowledge and the unstoppable perseverance born from overcoming hardship."[30]

My interpretation of Collins' message to "survive failure" is that a perceived failure is an opportunity to learn something. So, if you "fail" or make an error, pay attention to what you can learn instead of feeling defeated. I put the word "fail" in quotes because it isn't much a failure if you actually learn from it. However, if errors result in you feeling defeated, you may shy away from similar situations and you will then lose out on future learning opportunities.

Fostering resilience in the face of errors will not only help you learn medicine, it will also make it easier to handle some of the frustrating social aspects of training.[31] Consider when attendings "haze" you, questioning you on medical knowledge. If you are someone who is visibly afraid to fail, trembling when confronted, you will likely be the target of frequent hazing.

Conversely, if you explain that you don't know an answer without fear and behave confidently, you are less likely to be frequently picked on for questioning. I am not certain exactly why this tends to be the case, but I think of these scenarios as analogous to kids playing in the sandbox. Think about how a bully gives up teasing a kid who seems unaffected by it, but repeatedly taunts the kid who cries in response. Unfortunately, residency is a lot like the schoolyard.

One word of caution here: don't appear as if you don't give a damn about anything. Exude a persona that moves on relatively quickly from an error or potentially embarrassing mistake, but who is also dedicated to learning from a deficiency in knowledge or skill.

In sum, the more you embrace "failure" (or at least making errors) as an inevitable part of training, the less likely you are to perceive the experience negatively and the more you open up to learning opportunities that lead to you becoming an outstanding physician.

3. Practice mindfulness. What does it mean to practice mindfulness? Be aware of your mental, emotional, and physical state so that you can remain in control. Otherwise, physical or emotional discomfort can easily overwhelm the brain's deliberate cognitive functions, and this will affect clinical decisions.[32]

Consider one literal example of the power of the emotional brain: a stroke patient with facial paralysis is unable to activate a symmetric smile volitionally (when asked), but is amply capable when laughing at a funny joke. The latter action is controlled by the anterior cingulate, rather than cortically.[33] In this example, it is a pleasant surprise to witness the emotional brain "take over" and preserve an important human behavior. However, when it comes to making clinical decisions, you don't want emotional responses leading the way.

Some common distractions from on-shift tasks include hunger, a fight with a significant other, or news that a family member is ill. As long as you are self-aware of these potential distractions, you have the opportunity to handle the related feelings appropriately.

Before you start being short or crass with patients because you're "hangry," reach into that prepared snack bag. Before you let your mind wander to distracting personal matters, mentally shelve them as you walk into the hospital. Maybe you need to vent to a friend before a shift. However you decide to handle potential distractions, make sure you regularly check in with yourself in order to prevent negatively impacting patients.

I let emotion get the best of me once when I yelled at a respiratory therapist (RT), because I was so extremely anxious about an emergent pediatric intubation. "Get that stylet in the ET tube!" If I could go back, I would have been cognizant of physical manifestations of anxiety, like my rising heart rate, tense body posturing, and facial expressions. I would focus on getting a mental grip, slowing my mind, and calming my tone of voice. Then, I could have supported that RT by asking if she needed help, or implored others kindly to assist.

Again, whatever the scenario, the sooner you catch your mental distractions and find an outlet for them before letting them dictate your professional behavior, the better your clinical decisions will be.

The final example that underscores the importance of mindfulness comes from a struggling emergency medicine resident I know well. In their case, anxiety became a crippling barrier to professional growth. They regularly struggled on-shift with anxiety that they ascribed to "the great responsibility of not missing critical diagnoses (i.e., coronary syndromes) while having the wisdom of not overreacting to all potentially life-threatening complaints (i.e., chest pain that is actually muscular)."

This is one of the great challenges physicians face, especially in emergency medicine: to be thorough enough to not miss important diagnoses while not exposing patients to over-testing. Such a statement from this resident shows self-reflection, the precursor to practicing mindfulness. After identifying the source of the problem (anxiety about their ability to strike a balance in their practice), this resident followed steps to allow them to correct their actions and succeed in residency—namely, anxiety-reducing activities including meditation and therapy, and more rigorous studies that pertain to distinguishing limb- and life-threatening problems from red herrings.

The bottom line is that if you take a mindfulness approach to your own well-being, the care you deliver will be better because excellent clinical outcomes result from calculated and rational decisions, not emotional or reactive ones.

To those who say that the "gut" instinct is indeed valuable: emotionally based quick decisions are actually rooted in extensive experience engaging in critical thinking about the relevant subject or problem.[34]

The practice of mindfulness will serve you in and outside of your professional life. If you are interested in further reading on how human emotion relates to behavior, I suggest the elegantly written *Descartes' Error: Emotion, Reason, and the Human Brain* by Antonio Demasio.[35]

One final word on self-awareness with respect to those physically around you: *be cautious about what you say,* because you never know who is lurking around the corner—it could be a patient, a colleague, or a supervisor. In short, choose your words as if the room was crowded and everyone is listening. By making the conscious decision to bring a certain persona to work—not making particularly racy jokes, for example—you will never be caught saying something you shouldn't have.

I used to think that this meant giving up part of my character because I have, by some standards, a vulgar sense of humor. But it does not, it just means making a conscious decision to separate personal and professional life, and protecting your professional reputation

If you know an entire group of residents extraordinarily well, and you choose to do so, you can push the boundaries of the typical workplace conversation. But note that because you will be either rotating into other departments, or other specialty rotators will be rotating through your department, you run a risk of offending someone, and the result can be a tarnished reputation. I am not saying you should become a bore, just be aware of this information and use your discretion.

4. Maintain composure. Patients (and your team members) expect you to function at the same level during the first and last ten minutes of your shift, no matter what is going on in your life or how complex your other patients are.[36] This means that toward the end of shift, you should be highly attentive, composed, and not rushed. If you do rush or lose focus at the end of a shift because of fatigue, an emotional case, a desire to get home to your family, or any other reason, you will be more likely to cause an error.

I recall one Christmas Eve shift at Brigham and Women's Hospital having to tell a large family that their teenager passed away by a gunshot wound to the head. After crying in the bathroom for maybe forty-five seconds, I went back to my station and was reminded by a nurse that "the patient in Room Three had "been waiting quite a while" (though I recall this nurse also provided a qualifier that she "knows I had a tough case"). At that time, the idea of composing my mind to continue a long emergency department shift was daunting, but I had to for the rest of my patients. You will also be faced with maintaining composure after challenging cases and busy shifts.

There is no one perfect recipe for fostering resilience to traumatic events or exhaustion. However, I'd like to offer a few suggestions: First, practice enhanced mindfulness toward the end of a shift and after challenging cases. If you feel unable to concentrate, ask your supervisor for a break.

One strategy to safeguard against a rushed, uncomposed mental state at the end of a shift is to give yourself more time, and decide early in training that you accept that you will stay late, something like an hour past all shifts. This allows you ample time to "tuck in" all your patients, completing tasks and procedures and creating a well-thought-out plan to sign out to a co-resident. Tucking in your patients with plans that are straightforward is invaluable because the new team you sign out to will likely have to focus on seeing new patients, on top of caring for those already on the patient list.

An important side note about signing out a procedure: If you happen to know the resident coming on shift and that they have been seeking more experience with that particular procedure, you can sign it out. Just beware that you may upset the team if it is a busy day and you are essentially passing more work to the oncoming team. This is why signing out a procedure is generally a faux pas.

If for any reason you are stuck passing on a procedure for your workup or disposition plan during sign-out, then have a clear "if x, then y" plan. For example, "once the paracentesis is done and peritoneal fluid analysis comes back, decide on antibiotics and then send them to the medicine floor."

Another important aside, on rushing: there is a real and important distinction between *rushing* and *moving quickly* when the situation calls for it, such as seeing patients expeditiously when there is a busy waiting room in the emergency department. The main difference between the two is the rushed person typically *feels* and *behaves* flustered.

A final pointer on staying composed and focused: avoid too much socializing, otherwise, you run the risk of being viewed as someone who is distractible and unprofessional.[37] I don't suggest being a cold, robotic colleague who shuts down coworkers' attempts to be friendly. You can choose moments to engage in meaningful conversation, but it should not dominate your on-shift personality.

A suggested response if hospital staff attempts to engage with you when you have a long list of items to accomplish: "I would love to talk to you more about this after work." Find your own way to respond that fits your character. Doing so will give you the reputation as someone who is engaged and focused during work.

If you are able to stay composed throughout a shift, you will be free of fear that you missed something important. Leaving a shift confident that you did an excellent job, you position yourself to go home with the mental bandwidth to take on life outside the hospital: a side project in academics, the arts, or wherever your intrigue takes you.

5. Listen and provide feedback carefully during sign-out and team huddles. Any time your junior and senior residents speak, listen attentively to learn from their experience and mistakes.

Your colleagues share valuable information at sign-out in the form of clinical decision-making. Pay attention to what the attendings praise or criticize in other residents. This is key to getting excellent evaluations and fostering clinical critical thinking skills.

If, after listening closely to a colleague, you decide to give feedback, you should first consider asking yourself, "Is this person ready for the criticism?" How do you determine this? It depends on your relationship with the resident, who else is physically present, and the severity of the potential mistake.

An intern who you know well and is directly signing out to you will usually be open to your suggestions, for example, on antibiotic broadening for an immunocompromised patient. That same intern who is still your friend, but is now standing before a group of residents, medical students, and attendings, probably doesn't want to be corrected in front of the group by someone at their same level of training, regardless of how friendly you are.

In this case, make your point in private to avoid embarrassing them and to show that you are supportive and non-competitive. However, you are not doing the patient (or the resident), any favors by letting egregious mistakes go unnoticed, so speak up, and do so in a timely manner if you have a concern that delaying the feedback will cause patient harm.

One demonstrated effective strategy is hinting at suggestions through questions.[38] For example, instead of offering a different antibiotic choice, ask if there might be another option to consider.

6. Own your level of training. Foster the perspective that it is acceptable not to know something. With more experience, there should be less that you don't know, but you will always be learning new information and skills.

It is also true that information can come from the bottom up, and providers of all levels can offer something. Even a measly medical student can correct an attending on occasion.[39] Sometimes patients also have good suggestions, and we should heed them.

Own your level of training in part through your labeling yourself in an introduction. Such as: "Hi, I'm Dr. Richard Morty, *the first-year internal medicine resident.*" This is part of setting patients' expectations that is critical to the therapeutic relationship.

You can and should still behave confidently as an intern or at any junior stage, as this is important for patients' comfort. It is, however, important to strike a balance between self-assurance and communicating candidly about your level of experience. If you try to practice outside of your training level, you can cause poor patient outcomes.[40]

For instance, you never want to embark on a procedure alone that you do not feel one hundred percent confident performing. A paracentesis, for example, while considered one of the most straightforward procedures, is only straightforward *until* you hit an abdominal artery.

If you commit a major medical error, you will have to involve your supervisor and acknowledge the error with the patient and apologize.[41] (Although you probably won't be in apology mode right away if you hit the inferior epigastric artery).

With errors being inevitable, you should have an approach to dealing with them. Even something as simple as when a suture pulls through, apologize and acknowledge your mistake. This is a way to display honesty and integrity, and your patient and team will consequently trust you more.[42]

7. Have humility during successes and saves. Residents who are humble are more appreciated and admired than those who tend to gloat.

Humility is one of the most heavily weighted personal characteristics in managing impressions in the workplace, according to strong evidence provided by Bourdage, et al., out of the Department of Psychology at the University of Calgary. They found that those with more humility were less likely to require impression-managing behaviors with colleagues.[43]

So, when you get an IV the nurse can't or you obtain ROSC on a patient, don't point out your success, don't gloat, simply let the action be observed.

8. Maintain a balanced civilian life, with a focus on hobbies and organization outside work. According to HAEMR's newest assistant program director, Eric Shappell, the most successful residents tend to maintain significant interests outside residency: from regular family outings or camping trips to more ambitious projects like developing medical devices.

Those who find it challenging to maintain an outside interest should make time-budgeting and organizational adjustments.

To stay organized, keep a calendar and a notebook in your pocket with a to-do list you can constantly update. Or use a digital organizer, like Calendly or whatever app you prefer.

Finally, a word on financial organization: part of balancing civilian life is creating an operationally sound financial plan. Early in training find an excellent referral for two types of professional consultants: a financial planner and a certified public accountant (CPA).*[44]

---

* If you want a succinct text to help with loans, find Dr. Shappell's MD in the Black: A Personal Finance Curriculum for Residents.

9. Be as involved as possible in your program. This means regularly going to program events, including conferences, and, if possible, taking part in some form of quality improvement project. By doing these things, you will be appreciated for improving the brand under which you operate.

I used to think that going to residency events would put me at risk of being cornered socially and bored. But I realized after putting myself in these situations that while boredom may strike, plenty of awesome people and conversations happen in these settings as well. I wish I had made it to every possible gathering to have gotten to know my team better and express how much I valued my place in it.

1. Enjoy the process.

2. Accept failure.

3. Practice mindfulness.

4. Maintain composure.

5. Listen and provide feedback carefully during sign-out and team huddles.

6. Own your level of training.

7. Have humility during successes and saves.

8. Maintain a balanced civilian life, with a focus on hobbies and organization outside work.

9. Be as involved as possible in your program.

If you follow these nine recommendations you can hopefully maintain mental health throughout your training, and, if you master them, will make you standout clinicians as well. Now that we have covered the most important general recommendations, let's get into more specific scenarios and techniques that offer the most potential for you to demonstrate clinical competence.

9

Bedside Manner and Reassessment Approaches

How you enter a patient's room and introduce yourself sets the stage for how you are perceived as a physician. You need to learn to read a room and tailor your approach to each situation, however, I recommend consistently making the following considerations.

Even before you enter a room, be mindful of how composed you are. If you recently had a challenging clinical situation, especially a patient death, remind yourself before entering the next patient's room that each patient deserves your best.

To summarize one of my most supportive residency mentors at Massachusetts General Hospital,

Dr. David Peak: Every patient expects you to be equally thorough. The next patient you see doesn't care about the last person you saw or how complicated they were. The only thing they care about is what you are going to do for them—how you will take care of them.

If you perform a mental check and find yourself uncentered, or not fully prepared to give one hundred percent, take a moment to compose yourself. If needed, ask for coverage, so you can take a short break to recalibrate.

After you have effectively done this mental check, as you enter a patient room, greet everyone, not only the patient, but also their family, friends, and caregivers individually.

Place confidence and kindness in your tone as you introduce yourself in a manner that identifies what level of training you are in. Again, by "owning your position in training," you are forthcoming, building trust, and setting expectations that there is another physician supervisor backing your decisions. For example: "Hi, I'm Dr. Miguez, I'm the second-year internal medicine doctor on the team."

Next, consider acknowledging the patient's illness with something like, "I am sorry you are in the hospital." It is important to start with a brief supportive statement to align your interests with their speedy recovery.

Then, take a moment to consider making physical contact with the patient, as long as you deem it appropriate. If the anxiety from the COVID-19 pandemic has not yet simmered, consider avoiding contact altogether.

If things have calmed down, a hand on the shoulder or a handshake with your other hand covering theirs, for example, is powerful. There is something immensely therapeutic about human touch; it has been shown to facilitate trust in relationships, with proposed physiologic mechanisms varying from regulation of the oxytocinergic system in supporting social affiliation to rises in immune biomarkers.[45] Among oncologic patients, therapeutic touch has been shown to improve numerous pain-related parameters, including general activity, mood, walking ability, and sleep.

In addition to touch, eye contact has been shown among nurse-patient relationships to positively impact patient perceptions of care.[46] So, make sure to favor eye contact over staring at your computer or notepad. As discussed above, there is also evidence that interviewing a patient from a seated position improves patient satisfaction, in part by lengthening the perceived time spent with them.

Regardless of whether you choose to sit or stand, it is important to appear comfortable. However, don't be too casual. As friendly as patients want to be with you, they generally want a physician who maintains utmost *professionalism*, which includes everything from posture to language style. For example, I once heard from a resident that they received feedback from a patient for being "too casual" because they leaned on the wall of the room while interviewing them. Try to avoid this or any other posture that conveys a lackadaisical approach.

Similarly, avoid overly casual language, like a tendency I have to say, "hey, man" or "hey, dude." Some exceptions might be with teenagers or certain personality types, but you will have to gauge this cautiously at the risk of being seen in an unprofessional light.

REASSESSMENT APPROACHES

Pay special attention to how you approach reassessments because every patient interaction has immense potential to influence their perception of you. Each time you return to visit a patient's room you also can obtain invaluable data points that reflect their clinical trajectory, so that you can predict improvement or deterioration.[47] As such, I will elaborate on what I consider to be the most valuable components of a reassessment, including how to plan them, manage patient expectations, and budget time in each room.

How to plan reassessment. How you plan your reassessments depends on departmental type and census (essentially how busy the department is at that time). Consider how time-budgeting varies between a busy and slow day, or between an emergency department and a psychiatric ward.

During an emergency department shift with many high-acuity patients who need extensive physician monitoring, plan on "bouncing between rooms," frequently but rapidly laying eyes on patients to ensure you are at least gathering a gestalt of their clinical status.

Now, consider the locked psychiatry ward, where going in and out of rooms is practically more challenging and frequency of visits are limited. Here, focus on preparing a more comprehensive, singular "stop" to discuss all treatment options. This may mean spending more time reviewing their chart and discussing the plan with your supervisor in more detail before you start your reassessment.

How to manage patient expectations. Whether you plan on bouncing between rooms quickly or spending half an hour with each patient, you should set expectations early, and let patients know approximately how much time you will have to spend with them. For example, try telling a patient in broad strokes, "I am going to have to give a brief update, and I will return to discuss the plan in more detail shortly." Or "let's have a brief listen to your lungs, and I will return again shortly." By managing patient expectations of your visit, you buy extra time to return without them building frustration.

Further, during reassessments be efficient by consolidating tasks. For instance, you can re-auscultate a patient's lungs after their first round of a nebulizer treatment and follow this up with delivering X-ray results, all in a single reassess. Patients will appreciate your time efficiency.

How to budget time. If you are very limited on time, limit your reassessment to what is most relevant to why they are in the hospital: an abdominal re-examination if they presented for abdominal pain or a neurologic exam if they presented with focal numbness. And when patients try to keep you to ask questions, make sure to politely ask them to provide you additional time to reassess all of your other patients before returning to get into details.

The reassessment, in addition to creating an opportunity for patient appreciation of your time efficiency, is invaluable for obtaining a snapshot of patients' clinical status, through a quick view of their general appearance, vitals, and focused examination. In an instant, you have answers to questions like: How distressed are they? Were they more or less distressed than ten minutes ago?

You may find that answers to these questions relieves some cognitive burden by reducing anxiety of that feeling that you do not know how your patients are doing. You also are more likely to predict clinical decline and get ahead of it, because you will have a mental roadmap created from multiple patient visits.

10

Distinguishing Sick
from Not Sick

In all specialties, but particularly emergency med-icine, residents are evaluated on their ability to triage, or prioritize, different patients, and how they respond accordingly. The most challenging part of triage is consistently identifying "sick" patients, those with a high mortality risk, *when they appear well at first glance.* Consider pediatric patients who often look okay until the moment they cardiac arrest.

It is equally important to identify patients who appear ill but who are actually "not sick," in terms of new mortality risk (i.e., they're always chronically ill with a relatively high short-term mortality). These patients may have objective vital or lab data that are far from normal, but they don't merit immediate action because they are stable (their clinical trajectory is unlikely to change suddenly), and the "sick" patients need you more.

Consider the COPDer with an oxygen saturation of 89% on room air who is standing and breathing comfortably, because that is their baseline. Other examples will abound during training when you believe a patient needs immediate attention (based on the vital sign, lab value, or otherwise) but the attending or senior resident is not as concerned.

The converse will also happen early in training, when you find yourself wondering why an attending is concerned about a patient who appears to be in good health and relatively stable. They know something you don't. I will elaborate on *what* they know below.

But first, to answer a question I often hear residents ask, "How is it possible to be *too* concerned about a patient?"

Well, being too worried or worked up about a patient is a sign of missing the clinical point, poor clinical judgement, or a waste of cognitive energy (yes, you only have so much in a given day). It can be very annoying and time-consuming to deal with a resident who is overcome with worry about most of their patients.

And even in critically ill or coding patients, it never helps to panic. It always benefits the team and the patient to stay calm. You can still think and move expeditiously while maintaining mental and physical composure that bolsters team confidence.

So, what makes someone skillful at separating sick from not sick? A combination of experience and knowledge.

Interestingly, if you look at data on emergency department nurses' triage-decision accuracy, knowledge can be even more important for distinguishing sick from not sick than experience. Still, data from clinical trials and virtual simulations of emergency medicine triage suggests that the more time you spend with real-life clinical experiences, the more efficient you become in triage and hospital dispositions, which also happens to lower patient wait times and providers' work-related stress.[48]

The main message is that one can certainly improve upon their clinical competence in IDing truly sick patients by building a strong knowledge base. As such, I recommend that all residents focus on regular and rigorous study habits. I'm especially fond of question banks as they tend to be engaging, thus consolidating knowledge efficiently[49] and highlighting what is most relevant.

Specifc strategies to hone triage skills, that come from both my mentors and personal experience, are below. I preface these recommendations with the following disclaimer: it is unknown exactly what the best recipe is. This is my best attempt to create a general guideline to identify "sick" out of a sea of "not sick."

1. Develop a mental checklist of risk factors per complaint.

2. Have specific vital signs cut-offs to determine "sick."

3. Carefully observe attendings triage.

1. Establish a mental checklist of *especially high-risk factors* for common chief complaints (CC) that suggest a life-threatening or morbid underlying process. If these risk factors are present in the setting of the chief complaint, presume they are "sick" until proven otherwise.

Sometimes these high-risk factors are gathered before you even see the patient, by quickly scanning the EMR. This means that if you see any of these special risk factors present in the EMR for the given chief complaint, you must see that patient immediately.

For instance, if you look at the EMR on your computer and notice a CC of *head strike* in a 98-year-old, but you don't go see them immediately, this can be a high-stakes mistake. In this case, the important risk factor on your mental checklist was that this patient is *elderly*. Given the elderly population's relatively shrunken brains and stretched subdural bridging veins, the risk for traumatic subdural hemorrhage is relatively high.

You should label these patients "sick" in your mind until you have reassuring information that comes from an exam or imaging. If you go bedside and make your assessment and discover a normal neurologic exam, a history that includes they actually bumped their head on a bookshelf, and their BP is normally hypertensive on a daily basis, then you can mentally deescalate their acuity. But until you interview and examine them, you don't know.

Establish basic mental checklists when considering different chief complaints, and then expand on them. Start with something for head trauma like:

+ Elderly

+ Anticoagulation

+ Hypertension

Then, as you become comfortable with your list, expand it to include a larger number of high-risk historical factors as well as exam findings:

+ Elderly

+ Anticoagulation

+ Hypertension

+ Mechanism of injury

+ Neurologic findings

+ Signs of basilar skull fracture

There will be, of course, additional caveats to your checklists, which you will learn over time. For example, the severity of hypertension is an important distinction in the case of head trauma.

In the case of shortness of breath, your mental checklist should start with something like:

+ Work of breathing

+ Oxygen saturation

+ Baseline oxygen saturation

+ Respiratory rate

2. Have specific vital sign cutoffs that heighten your level of concern for "sick."

It is essential to have a framework for vital sign (VS) numerical cutoffs that get you to stop what you are doing and see the patient immediately. For the sake of simplicity, I offer a binomial framework for adult patients that tells you either "yes, I need to go see that patient right now," or "it can wait." How long "it can wait" is a sliding scale which is outside the scope of this text. Please keep in mind that this is a guideline and careful delegation, case-by-case, is required.

Artificial intelligence systems might one day lead the way for the best sliding scales in triage as well as treatment decisions,[50] but their utility in integrating big data to produce measurable healthcare outcomes is limited.[51] For now, we have to extrapolate from existing papers, old-school style.

Consider one informative study out of UCLA evaluating discharge vital signs that predict read-mission within seven days.[52] In this study, time-of-discharge vitals with at least twice the odds of re-admission were:

HR > **101** beats/min
SBP < **97** mm Hg
02 < **92%** SpO2 on room air
Temp > **37.3** °C

This study shows us that discharging a patient with these specific cutoffs might be premature. It may also suggest values that should raise our suspicion for a "sick patient." However, these values might not be so low that they require immediate action. To help you decide when to stop everything and go see a patient based on vitals alone, some basic cutoffs that I suggest are:

HR **135** beats/min
SBP **90** mm Hg
RR **35** breaths/min

O2 **92%** SpO2 on room air

Temp: **104°** F

(Note that I am not covering cutoffs on the less commonly seen end of the pathologic spectrum, including bradycardia, hypertension, bradypnea, and hypothermia.)

Once you hit these values, something is probably seriously wrong with that patient. To wait more than a minute to see them is bad medicine, with only a few exceptions. One exception is an actually very medically stable, "not sick" paraplegic who seems "sick" because they are hypotensive, but actually lives with autonomic instability, and often SBPs in the 80s, most of his adult life.

Also don't forget that someone can still be "sick" with normal vitals. For example, a patient can be septic with a normal heartrate secondary to being on a beta-blocker. So while the cutoffs I supply provide a framework for approaching the distinction between sick versus not sick, you will learn more exceptions with more experience.

3. Carefully observe attendings triage. Pay close attention to more experienced physicians as they prioritize one case over another. Try to learn why they do so. Ask questions about what data points they considered when making triage-related decisions. Ask "What made you see that patient first?" or "What concerned you about them?"

Find out early on what criteria (specific vitals, labs, exam findings, etc.,) gets attendings of different specialties concerned and on their toes, so that you can learn to predict clinical decline pertaining to varied systems and get ahead of it.

A urologist is going to pay close attention to overnight urine output to assess the renal system, and a cardiologist will consistently and carefully analyze his patients' daily ECGs to monitor heart health. The lesson here is simple: pay close attention to what your attending is worried about, and you are likely to take better care of your patients, as well as please your attendings. If you are rounding on a cardiac floor, focus your energy on items related to cardiology, like the ECG, troponin, pro-BNP, electrolytes, etc. This will demonstrate your appropriate focus on your patients' most relevant problems.

It may seem obvious, but you need to learn to focus on what your attendings are looking for. And this will most often depend on the simple fact of what specialty you are working with that day.

Also be aware that as you rotate through different teams and departments, you will find that the on-service attendings all have varying practice styles and levels of comfort with high-acuity patients.[53] More specifically, vital sign cutoffs that trigger alarm are going to vary widely by attending, and you should pay close attention to these idiosyncrasies in order to match your approach. Otherwise, your management of patients will differ from that of your attendings, and this won't reflect well in your evaluations.

HOW TO RESPOND TO "SICK"

So far, I have given tips on identifying sick patients, but not yet on how to respond to them. This is because it is usually obvious: Get help and start treatments based on guidelines you can find online, in UpToDate, or elsewhere. However, I have a few additional tips to guide you with treating the "sick" patient.

First, when you are seriously worried about a patient, *be high energy*. Not "energy" in the metaphysical sense, but commit your physical and mental drive to the case. How quickly you perform tasks and how carefully you think about the case can save lives.

With sick patients, you will move quickly to start the workup and treatment steps like obtaining IV access, sending off labs, performing an ECG, or calling for back-up, including your attending and consultants. You will also ultimately end up thinking much more about these cases, spending proportionally more time with them at the bedside than your other patients so you don't miss an important part of their history or exam. You should spend extra time performing a detailed examination and looking through their charts to learn about their medical and surgical history *intimately*.

Consider a patient you determine to be in septic shock but whom you don't have a source of infection. In this case, you need to go to the bedside immediately and look that patient over with a fine-toothed comb. They need to be rolled and every piece of skin on them examined for cellulitis. You also need to go through their medical chart in detail and look to see each procedure that they recently had that could be related to a culprit organism. Maybe you find after careful review of the chart that the patient had a dental extraction in the recent past, and this leads you to find a dental abscess on exam that needs drainage, which would have otherwise gone unnoticed.

In addition to being high energy, when you're a junior and identify a sick patient, **you have a responsibility to *get backup immediately.*** This means simply telling your nurse and attending that you are worried about a specific patient. It actually carries weight when you verbalize it: "I am worried about this one."

If you are a senior resident who is comfortable managing the patient's problem independently (or at least the first few steps of management, like starting fluids for hypotension), you are afforded a little time before getting backup. But this really depends on the culture of the program you are in, and in most cases, you should at least let your attending know someone is in relative trouble.

How quickly mid-level residents, PGY2s and PGY3s should get backup with "sick" cases is a bit more nuanced, and it depends on identifying the *severity* of "sick."

Consider a case of a *very* sick patient with a heart rate of 140. Let's say you think the cause of tachycardia is dehydration, and so you independently start administering fluids. But three liters of normal saline and an hour later, the heartrate hasn't changed, and you still have not asked for help. At this point, you are in trouble. The heart rate might be a cardiac dysrhythmia that you did not identify, and you may have put the patient in real danger by not getting backup earlier.

Conversely, let's say you have an adult asthmatic who presents with a *moderate* amount of wheezing. You decide to start albuterol nebulizers, and an hour later the wheezing has only slightly improved, but their oxygen saturation remains normal. Since your patient is not critically ill, and you have experience with asthma treatment, it may be reasonable to try more nebs and steroids before running and urgently getting your supervisors.

If you are ever uncertain and ask yourself *Should I bother my attending with this right now?*, the answer should always be *Yes*. This will protect your patients until you are more confident with your triage decisions.

Plenty of residents have been seen taking too long (with good intention, mind you) trying to get treatment started on their own, when they should have been getting backup to start taking the correct first steps.

Additionally, with sick patients, *how* you communicate to your team is important. Always maintain calm to avoid behaving flustered and transferring anxiety to your team or patient.

However, your word choice should convey gravity, especially when convincing a consultant specialist to urgently leave their home for the hospital. You may need to say something like, "This patient looks like they are about to code."

Getting backup from a consultant or team member can make the difference between a patient coding and stabilizing. Imagine you are caring for a patient with refractory cardiac chest pain, and you are getting pushback from your consulting interventional cardiologist on urgently coming into the hospital to perform PCI.

One reason consultants may be reluctant to act on what you say, jumping out of bed in the middle of the night and rushing into the hospital, is that you aren't doing a good job of communicating.[54] In this case, you are probably not communicating clearly the patient's *critical* illness.

11

Electronic Health Records (EHR): Documenting and Pre-rounding

Until the EHR gets a redo with complete integration of AI and powerful software that streamlines and automates notes, every resident should master EHR use, specifically with its use in pre-rounding and documentation.

To understand how major the EHR is in daily resident life, take a look at data from the STRIDE (Stanford Translational Research Integrated Database Environment) project, published by Wang and colleagues.[55] Over one hundred residents' use of the EHR was tracked between 2013 and 2016.

This led to analysis of over 15,000,000 unique EHR navigation actions.

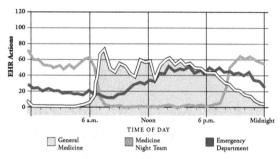

PGY1 Interns

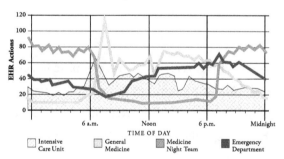

PGY2+ Residents

Mean number of EHR actions logged per user day in half-hour increments over a 24-hour cycle for different inpatient rotations, split by PGY1 interns (A) and PGY2+ residents (B).

EHR actions correspond to behaviors performed as clinicians navigate components (e.g. notes, orders, results) of a patient's chart.

PRE-ROUNDING

While seeing your patients for a focused exam before rounds is critical, it typically needs less explanation than how to prepare for rounds in other ways, including efficient chart review, focused learning, and time budgeting. In short, the most important steps to take when pre-rounding are:

1. Focus on the high points of the chart, like abnormal vitals and recent treatments.

2. Learn about and prepare to present on a topic relevant to a patient's diagnosis or treatment.

3. Give yourself ample time to pre-round, but don't start excessively early.

Let me first say that while on most department rotations, you will know which patients you will be assigned, and so you can pre-round by reviewing charts without difficulty. Sometimes, however, you don't know what patients you will be taking care of. Simply guessing which patients you are going to be caring for and then reviewing a pile of charts is not efficient or technically HIPAA compliant. However, if you plan to be participating in the patient care of your team's list in even a small way, it is HIPAA compliant and of immense practical application to look through the *high points* of their charts.

1. Focusing on the *high points* is my main tip for pre-rounding and review of charts. This means skimming all details and getting right to what matters, their chief complaint, *major* medical problems, *recent* vitals and labs, and *current* treatments. These pieces of information are what should be considered in decision-making on rounds. Most other details about a patient are usually superfluous.

Other *high points* to glean from the chart that will help you manage your list efficiently include identifying your sickest patients, as well as those who might be discharged. The former is essential in deciding which patients you spend the most time with, and the latter can facilitate expeditious discharges that will alleviate cognitive weight and reduce time spent on a patient that is ready for home.

2. The next tip on pre-rounding is to make time before you meet with your team to research a topic that is relevant to your current patient's disease process and treatment. It doesn't have to take more than fifteen or twenty minutes of your time to read a brief scientific article, watch a video on how to perform a procedure, review a picture that clarifies anatomy, or view a diagram that elucidates pathophysiology. Anything that you can share with your team will consolidate your learning and communicate a strong sense of professionalism.

For example, show up to rounds with several printed copies of a recently published paper within which you highlighted one or two sentences that summarize the main takeaway points. In thirty seconds, you can explain how that paper could be applied to your patient's care.

By doing things like briefly presenting a paper to your team, you have an opportunity to demonstrate skills in all of the six categories residency programs are told to assess by the Accreditation Council on Graduate Medical Education (ACGME) and The American Board of Medical Specialties (ABMS).[56]

+ Patient care and procedural skills. By sharing a paper, you are demonstrating care for patients through evidence-based practice.

+ Medical knowledge. You will garner this by regularly performing pre-round studies.

+ Practice-based learning and improvement. You can take what you learn to the bedside.

+ Interpersonal and communication skills. You have a chance to demonstrate these skills during your mini-presentation of a paper, diagram or video.

+ Professionalism. Demonstrating dedication to learning in your field is a key component of academic engagement and professionalism.

+ Systems-based practice. You can choose to focus on literature that critiques systems issues.

3. Finally, I would caution against one ubiquitous behavior among young trainees—waking up many hours before rounds, often at an ungodly hour, like 4:00 a.m., in order to prepare. If you spend hours pre-rounding, you will become less efficient from lack of sleep. The only potentially acceptable period to spend extra *hours* pre-rounding is in the first weeks of clinical rotations, when you are an early intern.

In *Why We Sleep*, Matthew Walker, the director of the Center for Human Sleep Science at UC Berkley, shows that productivity is dismantled by inadequate sleep—less than the seven to nine hours per night, according to the WHO. Such qualities that are affected by insufficient sleep include creativity, intelligence, motivation, effort, efficiency, collaboration, emotional stability, sociability, and honesty.[57]

If you tell yourself you are going to be a stellar resident by waking up before dawn to be "a master of chart details," memorizing the most you can about patients' histories, from every lab test and imaging study they have ever had to all of their medications and allergies, you will exhaust yourself, and without all-that-helpful data.

It's worth noting that knowing every detail of a patient chart neither applies to the ACGME or ABMS core criteria for evaluating residents. If a patient has a GI bleed, it's of no practical value to commit hemoglobin values to memory (which is time- and energy-consuming). It's more important to recognize when there has been a *drop of several points*. You will simply not be rewarded for spending hours reviewing charts, so why do it? If your hospital culture expects you to have all patient data at your fingertips, print them out or quickly jot them down, but do not try to commit them to memory.

DOCUMENTATION

While AI, speech recognition, and note documentation assist software from notable companies,
like Nuance and HealthNote, will soon make
my suggestions on documentation unnecessary,
for now we still have to focus on the strategies
that make this tedious, but ubiquitous, part of
training efficient.

The most important steps that I will elaborate
on below are:

1. Focus on quick, succinct notes.

2. Adapt *when* and *how* you choose to document based on what works in the given
   rotation.

3. Use technology to your advantage.

To justify writing quick notes over lengthy,
time-consuming ones, first let's consider the benefits
of longer notes.

The American Health Information Management Association (AHIMA) summarizes the benefits of detailed notes: coded data becomes quality reporting, physician report cards, and disease-tracking and trending, all of which translate into immense revenue through reimbursements.[58]

Another ostensible benefit to lengthy, eloquent notes: You can develop a reputation as a "great documenter."

Despite applications of coding data and the limited boost to your reputation as note king or queen, it is still vastly more important to focus on documenting *as quickly as possible* to optimize patient face-time. If you maximize your time at the bedside, comforting patients by answering their questions, you will deliver better care by creating more opportunities for communication. This also has the added benefit of reducing the likelihood of malpractice claims against you. As mentioned previously, when patients are interviewed about why they've sued their providers, they most often report feeling "unheard," and suits are typically closely tied to *poor communication.*[*]

Conversely, there is no good evidence that longer notes reduce malpractice claims.[59] Taking five minutes to bring your patient a blanket is a better use of your time than taking that time to add superfluous details to a note.

Finally, the likelihood you will save a life from behind your computer screen is low. And if you are ever going to "save a life" with documentation it is probably going to be along the lines of noting severe allergies and preventing a threatening medication from being given, which *only takes seconds* to document in the chart. Allergies *are* important, writing extensive details is not.

---

[*] The root causes of malpractice claims (in decreasing order) are misdiagnosis, procedural error, and medication or treatment error. While any of these claims could tangentially connect to a documentation error, this is a rare event according to the literature. See Schaffer, A. C., Jena, A. B., Seabury, S. A., Singh, H., Chalasani, V., & Kachalia, A. (2017). Rates and characteristics of paid malpractice claims among US physicians by specialty, 1992-2014. *JAMA Intern Med, 177*(5), 710.

With respect to *when* you choose to document, try varied strategies based on the service rotation you are on. Different rotations and departments will have different constraints that make certain documentation strategies a challenge. Consider how impractical it is to take notes immediately after seeing each patient in the emergency department, when patients are pouring in with high acuity. Notes need to be taken in batches after you have prioritized examining the patients presenting with potentially unstable conditions.

Experiment with taking notes in different ways, you might be surprised what works for you. I used to think that pulling up a patient chart in the room was grossly inefficient for me. I now realize that in the right setting, especially in a moderately busy pod, it can be very time-saving to open a note in the room (if there is a computer available) and type a few quick sentences into the H+P, place orders, or review relevant studies with a patient.

The strategy you choose will depend on several factors, including personal style and the department's patient acuity and volume. At different times, try documenting as you go, every two or three patients or in greater bulk, to figure out what works for you in varied clinical environments. You may even prefer to wait until the end of a shift to complete all of your notes.

Whatever strategy you adopt, I highly recommend jotting something down for each patient soon after you see them. This includes a brief past medical history and their presenting complaint, i.e. "56M with PMH of hypothyroidism here with one month of non-productive cough." Just enough so you remember them in a day or two if you have to go back. Do this so you don't end up looking back on a long list of other provider and nursing notes when trying to recollect anything about a patient.

To optimize technology for documenting, spend the time learning your system's macros, including for pulling laboratory data or imaging results into your notes. Also make macros for inserting phrases that you repeat in your notes four billion times a year. Relatively short time investments like a day or two taking a class with IT personnel will also save you tremendous time in the long run.

Finally, ask your tech-savvy colleagues what tricks they use. One of my co-residents brought a USB loaded with software that kept Epic from logging off so he never wasted time re-logging in to his computer. Brilliant.

12

Sign-out and Presenting

Feel free to skip this chapter on sign-out and presenting if you are a senior and you have this down pat.

Shift change sign-out is critically assessed by your colleagues and superiors, and will largely shape their impression of you.[60] Regardless of how informal sign-out appears, most everyone is paying attention to what you have to say.

As with attendings, most of the team is waiting to hear your *treatment plan*. Aspects of the treatment plan that are most important are speaking confidently and succinctly, in an organized manner, laying out a *crystal-clear* plan, and answering expected questions before they are even asked.

SPEAK CONFIDENTLY

A brief note on confident tone and posture when presenting. If you are able to convey confidence, this makes the incoming team feel at ease, reassured that there are excellent treatment plans (or workups) in place. The incoming team will feel relieved only having to pick up the slack in a few areas, so they can spend their energy seeing new patients.

Conversely, nothing is worse than when someone hands off a critically ill patient, and the provider sounds like they are unconfident and don't have a grasp on the underlying cause of illness or a treatment plan. That being said, you don't want to be disingenuous, claiming that you have a well-thought-out treatment plan when you actually don't.

If a patient's diagnosis or treatment plan is in the works, you can and should be forthcoming about this, prefacing your presentation by noting the patient is "undifferentiated" or "in need of more thought." This shows you are not afraid to ask for the team's help and that you are honest. However, every one of your patients cannot be "undifferentiated" with "unclear causes" and a "pending treatment plan." Repeating these phrases excessively will make you look lazy, incompetent, or both. Most of your patients should have a plan come sign-out time.

A WORD ON CONTENT

In terms of the content of your presentation, just be conscious that different providers will expect different degrees of thoroughness in your presentations. As long as you are aware of *the type of person* you are presenting to, you will be able to tailor your presentation appropriately. On identifying different styles of attendings and their preferences, see "Attendings and Directors" in Part I.

As a general rule, until you are familiar with the attending or team you are presenting to, it is safer to start with a more thorough presentation and then eventually whittle it down to bullet-point format. If you already know that the person receiving sign-out prefers brevity, give that.

With more experience, you will also provide less historic information and lab data at the start of each presentation, and spend more time getting right to *the plan*. Your discussion of a patient's treatment plan is really where you are critiqued most when you get beyond your intern year.

FOCUS ON MEDICATIONS

The focus in your plan should also typically be on *medications,* because this is what directly affects patients, in both directions—either contributing to a speedy recovery or contributing to mortality. The Institute of Medicine reports medication errors cause 1 out of 131 outpatient and 1 out of 854 inpatient deaths.*[61]

Thus, before rounds, perform regular mental checks that you are choosing and ordering (two distinct processes) the correct medications. You may want to consider discussing with pharmacy staff medication choices, dosages, and interactions before rounds. If one is available, pharmacy staff are invaluable resources who are often underutilized.[62] Also check and re-check in your computer system that what was ordered was correct.

Further, when it comes to presenting your plan (*with a focus on medications*), make sure you give a clear rationale for your decisions. For example, "Given Azithromycin covers most causes of

---

* In a 2014 review article by Dr. Christopher M. Wittich and colleagues of the Mayo Clinic, causes of medication errors are divided into healthcare professional-, patient-, and medication-related causes. The article also succinctly discusses the specific cognitive biases heightened at end of shift that can be especially detrimental to patient outcomes: confirmation bias (tendency to seek evidence supporting early hypotheses), lack of situational awareness, and cognitive errors. Please see Wittich, C. M., Burkle, C. M., & Lanier, W. L. (2014). Medication errors: An overview for clinicians. Mayo Clinic Proceedings, 89(8), 1116–1125.

community-acquired pneumonia, and the patient is well enough to go home, I chose this antibiotic." Or "Ciprofloxacin typically is what the patient improves on based on all of his past visits and culture data, so I chose this treatment."

DEPARTMENT STATUS AND PLAN

One final consideration prior to delving into a specific framework for sign-out presentations is departmental awareness (also the focus of the following chapter, but relevant here). This includes things like how many patients are in the department, how busy the waiting room is, and the patient list's general level of acuity (i.e., a long list of patients nearing ready for discharge versus all critically ill patients).

If you pay attention to how the overall department is doing in terms of things like capacity and acuity, you can tailor your presentation lengths accordingly. You will be immensely valued if on a busy day you speed up your sign-out, and if on a slower one, when you are afforded more opportunity for discussion, you provide more patient details and possibly even teaching points related to your cases.

Here is the format for signing out a patient and presenting:

1. Demographics (age, sex) and chief complaint with duration of symptoms

2. A brief history of present illness

3. Relevant vitals and exam findings

4. Relevant laboratory and imaging results

5. Assessment and plan

6. Disposition

1. Demographics (age, sex) and chief complaint with duration of symptoms

It is better for framing the problem to include chief complaint ahead of medical history (that alternative, listing medical history first, is a stone-aged and inefficient practice).

Consider the difference in these two examples: "Seventy-five-year-old male with two days of chest pain," as opposed to "Seventy-five-year-old male with past medical history of hypertension, diabetes, hyperthyroidism, anemia, hyperlipidemia, lung nodule, etc., who presents with two days of chest pain." Telling the team upfront the chief complaint frames what the team should be focusing on. If you are asked to change your format to state "the past medical" first, you can always do so.

As you become more familiar with this format (and as long as your sign-out receiver both trusts your clinical skills and appreciates brevity), you can present three quarters of an entire case in one short sentence, by simply adding diagnoses at the end. For example: "Mr. Levin is an eighty-year-old male presenting with chest pain for two weeks that is consistent with acute coronary syndrome." All you have to do now is add a plan.

2. A brief history of present illness

This is an area that often gets unnecessarily lengthy for juniors. Remember that the team can always ask for clarity and that you have taken a history in order to cherry-pick what you are going to convey as important historical items relevant to your assessment and plan. Different specialties will expect different content in your HPIs, however the principle is the same: **Provide only what supports your assessment and addresses expected questions or concerns.**

3. Relevant vitals and exam findings

Only abnormal vitals and exam findings should be reported. The major exception to this rule is very early on in training (i.e., early intern year) when you may be expected to robotically verbalize each normal vital and a comprehensive list of exam findings regardless of the chief complaint.

Later in training, you will learn which specific normal findings the team wants to hear about. For example, your presentation of a patient with a history of congestive heart failure who presents with shortness of breath that you believe is due to pneumonia, should not only include any adventitious lung sounds you heard, but also that there is "no jugular venous distension (JVD)" and "no lower extremity edema." This suggests you at least considered heart failure as a potential cause of shortness of breath.

The senior resident is more trusted, and fewer details of vitals and exam are needed to assure the attending that your assessments are generally accurate. As a reminder, you can learn exactly how much detail to provide to a specific attending and team by observing your co-residents and noting what is praised versus what is criticized.

4. Relevant laboratory and imaging results

The same conventions apply to lab and imaging results. *Offer only abnormal results* unless you are expected to be more thorough at your stage of training.

Also mention normal results when they are pertinent. If you are presenting a case of a GI bleed, briefly stating a normal hemoglobin will convey an understanding for what the team is waiting to hear. As with a GI bleed, different chief complaints will cause your sign-out team to listen for particular results.

A presentation on a case of blunt head trauma should include platelets, PT-INR and CAT scan results (even if they are normal). In septic patients, blood pressure, white count, lactate, and creatinine are most pertinent. As you gain clinical experience, you will solidify your understanding of what is or what is not relevant information for a given chief complaint or problem.

Finally, **get to the point and lead with profound information** even if it seems out of order. For example, skip reporting the CBC if you know that there is intracranial hemorrhage on a CAT scan of the head. You can report the platelet value later.

5. Assessment and plan

Mentally commit. Say out loud what you think the diagnosis is, and do it confidently. Stick to a simple, consistent statement like: "I think they have X."

It's better to be wrong than to constantly hedge, saying, "It could be anything, from X, Y, and Z to Ebola." Such indecisiveness can be appropriate for early interns, but won't serve your learning or evaluations soon thereafter.

Conversely, it is reasonable to include a differential of potential causes as long as you still **commit to a most-likely diagnosis** by saying something like, "I think they have X, but am also a little worried about Y and Z, and will rule them out with these studies."

While assessments are sometimes praised for candor when a senior resident is honest about not knowing the exact cause for a patient's illness, this is only in truly challenging, rare cases. Otherwise, it is unacceptable to say you don't have a relatively certain assessment of your patient. If you don't have a grasp on the under-lying cause of many of your patients' illnesses, leadership will begin to notice. Especially when you are a senior.

Finally, with your plan, *be as concise as possible.* As an intern, your attending probably wants to hear more information in the plan, including which specific labs you are going to order. But as you ascend, stick to only actionable items like imaging versus no imaging, and add your reasoning. Form a plan like this: "If study X is not revealing, then I will order Y, because if both are negative then we have ruled out all concerning etiologies, and they can follow up with their PCP." This is enough to convey mature, critical thinking.

6. Disposition

You will develop foresight of patients' dispositions with time. You should start concluding your presentations as an intern with a few words (and no more) about "dispo" and the reasoning for your choice. For example, "Hopefully in a day or two as long as he/she can maintain an oxygen saturation at 95% with ambulation, he/she can go home on PO antibiotics." With this example in mind, you should note that setting clear and objective cutoffs for your decisions (like oxygen saturation of 95 or above) will be highly valued by your team.

PITFALLS DURING SIGN-OUT

Finally, please be aware of the most common pitfalls during sign-out in order to avoid them:

1. An overly broad differential

2. Lack of confidence

3. Behaving distracted

4. Poor listening

5. Poor problem prioritization

6. Missing the big picture

1. An overly broad differential in attempt to exhibit your knowledge base.

This typically hurts you because it shows a lack of critical thinking. Your attendings and mentors want to see you decide on **a single diagnosis** or **a short differential** that is worth considering. Your supervisors may have you do mental exercises creating long differentials,[63] but, for the most part, attendings do not want you to recite a long list of possible causes of a chief complaint in your presentations at sign-out.

2. Lack of confidence.

Even on day one of rotations you need to find confidence in yourself so that you can perform well. More than a century ago, Arthur Bandura explained how self-confidence, defined as a person's judgement of his/her capability to perform, impacts motivation, effort, persistence, and eventual academic success.[64]

You won't be a highly competent physician right away, but don't let that shatter your confidence. Recall that before residency you harnessed confidence throughout an adult life of many achievements. When you speak, know that you are putting forth your best attempt given limited clinical experience.

3. Distractions.

Don't try and "tie up loose ends" or do patient care or notes on rounds unless there is a critical change in patient stability. When you are on rounds, focus on rounds.

4. Not listening or focusing on what your team is saying.

Don't be focused on internally reciting what you are going to say when your turn comes to present. It is a tough urge to fight. Be confident that you already know your patients. Every patient really requires only a few major points anyway: their short story, diagnosis, treatment, and disposition.

If you are listening to your team, you will learn from them, not just adding to your knowledge base, but you will learn different ways to think about cases, oratory styles, and lingos that you may like and decide to adopt.[65]

Also, pay close attention to your juniors' mistakes, the maturity of your seniors' presentations, and how each is similar to or different from your own style. This mental exercise will help you perfect sign-out communication.

5. Poor problem prioritization.

Residents will often make the mistake of focusing on the small fish. For example, discussing treatment of a patient's chief complaint of a cough, despite the patient having bigger problems that have been revealed through their work-up, like an acute ST-elevation myocardial infarction (MI) seen on ECG. In this case, the assessment and plan should be focused on treatment of the MI, not the cough. The patient has bigger fish to fry than a cough. Focus on the big fish.

6. Missing the big-picture plan.

Consider a well-intentioned intern who correctly diagnoses a one-hundred-year-old patient with an ST-elevation MI (STEMI). The intern adds in their plan the standard treatment for patients who have STEMI: calling cardiology for urgent catheterization. The problem is that they did not realize that the patient's grave disability or dementia will likely preclude them from heart catheterization. Not that one should not call cardiology, but the idea is that the patient will likely not be going for a major life-threatening procedure, given their baseline functional status. And if you present the case in a manner suggesting you are thinking the patient is going for a cath, you will have missed the big picture.

A more experienced resident tends to demonstrate awareness not only of the baseline functionality of patients, but also of the social and practical considerations important to their disposition: things like a safe travel plan home and the safety of the home environment. Consider a nine-year-old asthmatic who is no longer wheezing after you gave them nebulizers and steroids, and who can technically be medically discharged. But discharged under whose supervision? And does that person know how to work a nebulizer machine? If not, they need to be taught, or disposition needs to be reconsidered.

13

Departmental Awareness

This section is about your awareness of the microcosm that is your floor or department. You want to know your department inside and out, including *where equipment is, patient capacity, and bottlenecks to patient flow* through the department.

Why care about these specific departmental issues?

Knowing where equipment "lives" is important because when emergent procedures arise, you don't want to waste any time searching. When patients become unexpectedly unstable, seconds count, and you need to be *self-sufficient* in finding necessary equipment with *the option* of asking others to find something as a *back-up*.

With respect to knowledge of *patient capacity*, it is integral to demonstrate resident leadership. For instance, if you have a department with thirty patients filling all thirty of your beds, a resident who prioritizes discharges facilitates opening a bed to care for new patients. As does a resident who keeps an eye on the waiting room in the emergency department, picking up the pace when they notice that the total number waiting suddenly expanded. This person is seen as a mature physician with attention to systems issues.

An example of a bottleneck to "patient flow," or movement through the department, is the difficulty in *obtaining imaging results* from a radiologist. In this setting, a radiologist's reading of a chest X-ray might be the only thing keeping a patient from being moved out of the ER and admitted, or possibly going home.

If you are someone who learns where the bottlenecks are—obtaining imaging results, moving a patient between triage and their room for physician evaluation, or from patients' rooms to the imaging department—you can develop efficiency tricks (which I will explain below).

How does one learn where equipment is? Look.

I recommend showing up an hour or two early when you first begin a new work environment to look around. Open drawers to take your first look, so you don't have to do so in an emergency or search for things in front of a patient like you've never been there before. Rather, in front of the patients, you want to make it look like you are comfortable with where everything is: make it look like you live there, like you are an *actual* resident of the hospital.

How do you learn about patient capacity in real time? Ask.

If you're new to the department, ask your attending: How many beds do we have in the department? Or you could find this information online or by simply walking the department and counting beds.

Further, when coming on-shift to a rotation you've become familiar with, make it a habit to ask your team upon arrival: Who are potential discharges? If you don't have any critically ill patients, you can suggest presenting these "quick discharge" patients first to get them home-bound.

How do you learn about the bottlenecks in a particular department? Again, asking is probably your best bet: "What are the usual bottlenecks to flow and discharge here?"

If you asked me this question about any emergency department I've worked in, I would answer that typical bottlenecks to patient disposition are *imaging, consults, and procedures.* If you prioritize these, you will most expeditiously diagnose and treat patients, and then be able to move them out of the emergency department to in-patient status or discharge them.

How do you prioritize *these* specific bottlenecks?

Place orders for a study, and page a consultant as soon as you leave the patient's room. **Nothing else comes first** (unless someone under your care at that exact moment is critically ill). Also, start setting up for procedures as soon as you can allot the time to carry it out.

With the *imaging bottleneck,* it may not be as simple as *ordering the test* and assuming it will be done expeditiously. You have to stay on top of every stage of movement from the patient to the X-ray machine or CAT scanner.

Speak to the radiologist to protocol the study (basically giving approval for the test and exactly what modality they deem appropriate, like with or without contrast, etc.). Call the radiology technician to prioritize the patient in the queue. Speak with the transport personnel to come pick the patient up. Maybe you have to wheel or walk the patient to the imaging room yourself. Maybe you have to help the nurse obtain an IV that is a suitable caliber for the contrast study required.

Once the imaging has been performed, you might even have to call the radiologist to put in a preliminary "wet read," so you can get a general sense of what is going on. The point is, you have to act as a facilitator by paying attention to where specifically the hold-ups are, and problem-solve.

With regard to the *consult bottleneck* you need to be aware of a few things. First, before placing that immediate surgery consult the moment the patient arrives in your department, ask yourself: "If my workup is normal, will I still need the consult?" If the answer is yes, as in many recently post-operative patients, then you should place the consult upon the patient's arrival into your department.

There are many reasons why surgeons will want to be alerted that their post-op patients are arriving in the hospital despite a normal workup. For instance, they often will want to observe patients in-house to monitor for development of complications imaging and labs might not pick up; i.e., a micro-perforation that a CAT scan won't show but that could turn into a larger perforation.

If you think that you will be able to safely discharge the patient if your work-up and observation period is reassuring, then don't place the consult at all. Simply have the patient follow up with their surgeon or other specialist as an outpatient. You can still call the patient's surgeon to give them an FYI that their patient came to see you in the ED or wherever you're working, and let them know you don't feel they need to come see them, and are letting them know as a courtesy. Also, be aware that a courtesy call isn't always received as such, and some attendings may be bothered by a call that doesn't warrant them taking specific action.

Second, when calling consultants, know that they usually like to hear that the workup is in progress. This reassures them that you are not completely relying on them to manage *your* patient. To explain to consultants that the workup is underway, you can say something to the effect of: "The CT scan of the abdomen and pelvis with contrast is pending. I'll make sure it gets done quickly, and I can page you when it is done, or you can be on the lookout."

One caveat to starting workups on patients without consultant involvement has to do with *transplant patients*. Among these patients, their specialists often prefer you do little to nothing to the patient without talking to their team first, so place the call expeditiously.

As a reminder, never be timid with consultants. Ask for their name, politely, up front. This invokes accountability and makes them less likely to be a jerk. If they go beyond jerkish behavior and are completely inappropriate, cursing or yelling, respond matter-of-factly without emotional energy. Say something like, "I don't appreciate the way you are speaking to me."

Follow this up with solution-oriented, patient-care driven language. You will have to choose words depending on the case, but consider something like this. "Why don't you come see the patient? They will benefit from your expertise, and you can let me know what you think." Most consultants will have a difficult time refusing a consult so long as you express a desire for their expertise and specify your concerns.

14

Academic Engagement

Academic engagement here refers more to how to *approach* learning, rather than the *content* of what you study.

Active learning is the most valuable approach, and it includes things like going to conferences and *asking questions, participating* in simulation labs, and *on-shift reading* about research that is *relevant* to your patients' treatments. This is opposed to more *passive* learning, like reading a chapter in a textbook daily.

You can still read up on a subject you are relatively uncomfortable with, but you should budget your time to focus on more engaging activities. The knowledge consolidated from challenging patient cases and simulation labs is far more substantial than reading chapters or sitting in the back of a lecture hall occasionally listening to the speaker.

Q-BANKS

You can *actively* learn in preparation for your clinical duties with *mentally-engaging* study practices, especially by doing question banks (Q-banks), and focusing on subjects you are relatively deficient in. Q-banks augment memory consolidation of medical knowledge through the challenge and engagement of question format.

When you work with Q-banks, use the software's filters to **spend time on subjects you feel relatively uncomfortable with.** If you need a deeper understanding of the concept, you can supplement Q-banks with a textbook, but the majority of these Q-banks will already include in-depth explanations.

PRETEND MAKING SOLO DECISIONS

During clinic duties, the most valuable way to improve your knowledge base is to pretend you are the only physician available (i.e., you have no attending or resident back-up). The more you feel like you have real responsibility for your patients, that your decisions matter and affect patient care, the sooner you will make leaps in learning and clinical competence. Why does this happen? Because when information carries significance, it will be consolidated into memory more efficiently. If you feel your decisions are important, you will also more regularly carve out study time.

This heightened sense of responsibility affects residents' clinical capability. It is evident in the major leaps that residents make right around when they transition from first-year residents to second-year, second to third, and so on.

You can "trick your mind" into feeling this sense of responsibility at any time, by basically pretending you are on your own. This means that before you present a case to your attending, you will have thought about your differential diagnoses, workup, and treatment plan as an *independent provider*. After discussing with your attending, consider what would have been missed or potentially gone wrong if you did not have them there to correct you. Part of training is, of course, to have the attending teach you. But start trying to separate yourself from the mental crutch of knowing someone is there to help you, and you will more readily become a capable resident.

CLOSELY OBSERVE CO-RESIDENTS

Another way to engage with your education in a productive manner is to closely observe your co-residents' actions and decisions on-shift—both successes and mistakes. You can adopt helpful strategies and avoid repeating their mistakes.

I remember watching a co-resident start to treat ischemic chest pain with nitroglycerin in the case of an inferior-MI, without checking first to see if there might be right ventricular (RV) involvement, with a right-sided ECG. That patient became hypotensive and almost arrested because they in fact had RV involvement. The attending grilled the resident. By starting to check R-sided ECGs in all inferior MIs, I avoided the mistake and potential patient harm.

One caveat to learning from observing your co-residents is that if you are an intern, it might feel daunting to try and adopt the strategies of a fourth-year resident. This is because you are at a completely different stage of training. As such, you might choose to pay more attention to residents a year above you, rather than three or four, when looking to adopt new clinical strategies.

END-OF-SHIFT REFLECTION

Finally, routinely ask yourself at the end of every shift how you can improve in order to fill in your knowledge gaps and optimize general, systematic issues, like your ability to see as many patients as your co-residents.

It will be easier to identify *specific* gaps in knowledge than your *general* weaknesses, especially if the latter are tied to personality traits, like stubbornness. It is easier for a person to say, "I just don't know the dose of that medication" than "I really don't know how to manage a patient list." The second example might pose an insult to personal ego, making it harder to acknowledge. As a reminder, in order to prevent ego from hampering your improvement as a trainee, you need to allow for frequent failure, and not let it affect your sense of self-worth.

If you are able to push ego aside, and be honest with yourself about your shortcomings, you will be able to make significant improvements to your practice. For example, if you are able to accept that you are disorganized in your presentations on rounds, you can take the next corrective step, *figure out why*. You might do so by analyzing how organized presenters work. It might be that these highly organized residents have concise and appropriate treatment plans on rounds for the simple reason that they only take on a few patients at a time. Maybe you need to limit the number of patients you are taking on until you feel comfortable with the workload. In doing so, you might also find that fewer patients translates to better, more organized presentations, because you have given yourself more time to think about each case.

15

Death and Dying

Dealing with death and dying as a trainee may be one of the most challenging experiences of your life. In order to be prepared, it is critical to strategize for the following steps: discussing goals of care questions with patients, family, and healthcare proxies; sharing your prognoses with the critically ill; employing end-of-life care that maintains dignity and optimizes comfort; and breaking horrific news in the immediate aftermath of losing a patient.

GOALS OF CARE DISCUSSION

One of the reasons it feels daunting as a young trainee to broach goals of care discussions with patients is that there is a very broad spectrum of patient preferences, from a patient choosing every imaginable treatment to sustain life, all the way to comfort measures only. Another reason, of course, is that this discussion is a completely novel experience for you.

While it may feel intimidating at first, if you focus on learning the *major components* of any goals of care (GOC) discussion, you will have a solid foundation to build upon. The major components are **CPR and intubation (or code status), medical aggressiveness, and procedural limitations.**

How to have the discussion?

When discussing all components of GOC, it is imperative to be especially mindful of your *tone*. Appropriate tone is essential for patients to feel adequately cared for. GOC discussions are often a sensitive subject for patients, so you want to carry a *serious* tone, while *not being ominous-sounding*. How serious do you need to sound? That depends on how critical the GOC discussion is at that time. Are you discussing the GOC for completion's sake, filling in part of their chart that has been absent, or because you are actually worried that they might code during their current hospital visit, and you expect it will drive management decisions?

Even if you aren't seriously worried they might code in the same visit, still remain cautious not to be blasé about the topic. While you may have asked these questions a thousand times before, it may be the first time the patient has considered them.

When should you have the discussion?

In addition to *tone, the timing of when* you broach GOC is of immense importance. Don't ask patients as soon as they enter a room: "What's your code status?" Try to wait for the appropriate time, toward the end of your encounter, making the questions seem like part of a standardized mental checklist you go through. Otherwise, you run the risk of scaring them.

What do you say?

Preface your interest in broaching the GOC discussion. For example, ". . . I also ask this of every patient I care for, from the youngest and healthiest to the most elderly and sick...and I don't expect this to be an issue today . . ."

And then ask, "If your heart were to stop for any reason, would you want CPR? If you were to stop breathing, would you want us to breathe for you, put you to sleep on a ventilator, until it can be safely removed?"

A common response to this latter question is, "How long will I be on a ventilator for?" I typically explain that *there is no crystal ball* as to whether they will be asleep on a ventilator for a day, a week, or longer. In all cases, you should provide your impression and clinical sense of whether intubation is temporary or, for all practical purposes, a dead end for them (like if they are in their late nineties with multiple severe chronic comorbidities).

If the patient is young and healthy with a severe asthma flair, they might only require a day or two of breathing assistance before a trial-of-extubation. In any case, your input regarding these details can be invaluable in helping patients make decisions that are consistent with their values. Without medical opinion, a patient can't reasonably decide on things like how much risk they want to take, or how much suffering they are willing to endure, for a chance at recovery.

Unfortunately, no matter how tactful you are in providing your opinion, you will still have patients who are unwilling to broach any part of a GOC discussion. This could be because such a discussion frightens them, or maybe it is culturally an off-topic matter. They may have had a bad previous in-hospital experience.

If they resist, you have two options: push a little, or let it go. If the patient is in no real danger of decompensating, defer the discussion to whenever they are mentally prepared. If a patient looks like they may arrest, however, you might want to tell them something like, "I know this is a very tough decision, I just would prefer to be able to have a planned discussion with you, rather than it be a sudden and rushed conversation. I certainly want your wishes to be clear if you are unable to speak for yourself." Pick any version of a statement that conveys urgency, while trying not to frighten them too much.

Finally, there are a few circumstances around code status discussions that should be brought to your attention, so you are not surprised when they occur:

1.   When to double-check documented code status.

2.   When a new patient is actively dying.

3.   When a healthcare proxy (HCP) changes a code status of an actively dying patient.

1. When to double-check code status.

If you're caring for a severely disabled person such as a one-hundred-year-old man who is bedbound and aphasic from prior strokes, and you see on record "FULL CODE," you should ask yourself is this accurate? While you should not place moral judgements on patients' choices, their computer-based code status may not be current (like if they have not seen a doctor in twenty years), or they may not fully understand what CPR or intubation actually is.

It would be in your patient's best interests to do a little more detective work on the subject. Maybe the patient is certain, at one hundred years old with multiple severe medical problems, that they want to be alive at all costs. But at least confirm with them or speak to a family member who is HCP about what CPR can entail—breaking multiple ribs, sometimes shocking the heart multiple times, etc.—if they are being seen again in the hospital for an acute problem. Providing them with accurate information about a procedure allows patients and healthcare proxies to make the most informed decisions.

Our job is never to coerce, so make sure to check yourself that you are not trying to impose your morals on your patients.

2. When a new patient who is dying arrives.

If a new patient presents to you actively dying, and they can't communicate (and no family is reachable), you may have to make a quick decision. Your decision may incorporate an attempt to obtain their POLST or advanced directive. Only spend a short time tracking down these documents. Recall that you can always remove life-sustaining treatment once you've tracked down their papers expressing goals of care, but you can't bring them back from the dead, so don't delay life-saving moves.

Consider a patient who arrives in severe respiratory distress, with an oxygen saturation of eighty percent on a non-rebreather, which is non-sustainable for life, or at least not without anoxic brain injury. In this case, you would need to prioritize getting that patient intubated. If you can access their code status in a moment (like if the EMS hands you an advanced directive), then you need to rapidly look at that information to determine whether or not you intubate. Otherwise, do the procedure, save their life, and then later figure out goals of care.

3. When an HCP changes code status of an actively dying patient.

If an HCP changes a patient's code status with a verbal order, while it poses a potential moral dilemma, you are generally legally obligated to abide their wishes. Two common exceptions include:

a. You believe a medical intervention to be futile in preserving a life. In these cases, you do not have to abide a HCP's wishes.[66]

b. You don't believe the HCP is truly acting as a surrogate for what the patient would want. Consider the case of a patient who you, or other providers in your department around you, know personally (from recurrent hospital visits or otherwise). The HCP's decision to change code status might seem inconsistent with everything the patient previously expressed. This is a very challenging circumstance and requires cautious action, especially to cover yourself legally.

The most important advice, not only from a legal protective stance, but also for patient advocacy, is to take a multidisciplinary approach that involves "legal" and your hospital's ethics committee.[67] Additionally, the patient's primary care physician and other specialists who know the patient should be contacted to obtain collateral information that might improve your understanding of their wishes. For example, it would be tremendously helpful to know that the primary care doctor just met with the patient and family a few days ago, and had an extensive conversation on goals of care.

If time allows, you may need to hold a meeting including the dying patient's family and your hospital's administration (including "legal"), in order to discuss final decision-making. Note that the administration's presence can partially shield you from potential legal trouble.

The final piece of advice here is: when you ask a HCP about their loved one's goals, it helps to specifically ask, "What would *they* [the patient] want?" Sometimes the answer reveals that the HCP is really afraid of losing their loved one, but are not acting on their behalf.

While you are certainly not expected to manage the most complex of these situations as an intern alone, it is invaluable to your development as a physician to be as involved as possible early in training. The last thing you want is to become a senior resident or attending that is inexperienced with such scenarios and conversations.

MEDICAL AND SURGICAL AGGRESSIVENESS

For patients at the end of life, due to age or chronic illness, you must establish if they want particular *classes of medicine*, as well as whether or not they would want *minor or major surgery*. There is a time and a place for internists and specialists to broach the details of this medication or that, one surgery versus another, but for the majority of your practice as a resident, knowing how aggressive to be in *a general sense,* will mostly suffice. One exception is if you are a surgery resident, you might want to know more details about patients' surgical preferences than what I suggest below.

First, find out whether they want the following classes of medications: **fluids, antibiotics, and vasopressors.** Even if you are not going to be managing vasopressors regularly, it is helpful to know if they would want pressors because this information can help you understand the patient's disposition throughout the hospital. Consider a patient who is gravely ill and who needs admission for septic shock and antibiotics. The decision to admit them to a general hospital bed versus the ICU often comes down to whether or not they would ever want a central line placed to receive vasopressors (recall you can only run vasopressors safely through a peripheral IV for a short time, on the order of a few hours).

Here are some sample questions to find out what classes of medications a patient wants: "So that I can get a sense of what types of treatments you want, would you want antibiotics? How about fluids? And blood-pressure-supporting medication (vasopressors)? This requires special placement of a central line, or a large IV into the neck or groin vein, and we place a catheter (or plastic tubing) that then goes near to the heart. This would mean you would need to go to an intensive care unit. Would you want this?"

Often you will be asked further details of the procedure, like how common it is and what the risks are, including pain level.

While you do not need to ask patients about every procedure they might need one day, it is generally good to know whether they would want any surgery. And, if so, how about *major* surgery like open laparotomy or neurosurgery? Or would they only want *minor* surgery like a small abscess incision and drainage?

HOSPITAL ADMISSION

Understanding a patient's thoughts on admission early in their hospital course will also help you prepare their treatment plan. Some patients are one-hundred-percent certain that they would never want to be admitted at their stage of life, while others want the so-called "full court press," ICU, and all possible life-sustaining treatments.

You can easily distinguish a patient's preferences by asking direct questions, including: "Would you want to be admitted?" If they respond "no," then you might need to consider asking this: "Are you aware that this illness could (or will likely) be fatal without in-hospital (like IV) treatments?"

If a patient agrees to be admitted, just as with the surgical decision, you want to tease out how aggressive to be in your admission plan, and ask clarifying questions like: "Are you okay going to an intensive care unit?" For some patients, the benefits of constant supervision by ICU nurses is outweighed by the discomfort of being bothered, or woken, every hour for vital sign checks.

DYING PATIENTS

When a patient is expected to pass away in the hospital based on their severity of illness, your focus becomes *preserving dignity and optimizing comfort*.

The best way to facilitate both dignity and comfort is to involve other teams in that patient's care, by placing consults to the following teams (as long as they are available), while you focus on medical management: palliative, pain, religious (chaplain, rabbi, etc.), and social work services. This kind of multidisciplinary approach can rarely be matched by an individual practitioner. First, you still typically have to continue with other patient responsibilities, but also because these services are administered by individuals with special training for handling these tough situations.

The palliative team will often help family members with challenging decisions and offer an array of suggestions for comfort-based medications.

The pain service can sometimes arrange for Patient Controlled Analgesic (PCA) pumps.

Religious figures can offer the bedside end-of-life goals that can individualize care.

Social work can help with a long list of things, including family planning for what happens with the patient's body (cremation, etc.), offering a space for the family to grieve, and safe travel arrangements.

In addition to a multidisciplinary approach, help maintain your patient's end-of-life dignity by creating a quiet, private environment. Make sure staff, including nurses, are aware that they should only enter the room when necessary to address patient comfort, and that noise should be kept to a minimum.

Continue therapies that are effective in short-term comfort like morphine, but remove extraneous lines like second IVs, BP cuffs, and cardiac and oxygen monitors that won't change management.

Finally, when you start to learn the indicators that suggest a patient is nearing death—labored breathing patterns and severe bradycardia—you can warn the patient's family that they are about to pass, and that this might be the last chance for them to be with their loved one. Once they pass, you will have to learn how to proclaim death, but I will leave that out of this text, as institutional requirements can vary.

BREAKING THE NEWS

If the family is not bedside when their loved one passes, but they arrive at the hospital later, you will have to break the terrible news, and you will again be reminded how challenging our job is.

In terms of where to begin, the best framework I've used is to *first find a private place,* and then **tell a brief story** that includes what happened upon presentation, the treatments you tried that failed, and then the outcome.

Imagine that a family comes in screaming, "Where is my baby!?!?" or "Is he dead!?!?"

It is more humane to tell the brief story than to bluntly answer, "He is dead," or "Yes, he's dead."

For example, "When he came in, he did not have a pulse, and he was not breathing. We attempted resuscitation for several hours, giving him multiple heart shocks and medications. After trying everything possible, we were unable to get him back, and, unfortunately, he passed away. I am so sorry."

These stories, describing the events that led to their death, help loved ones understand that you and your team did everything possible. A brief explanation does not prolong the anticipated answer too much, while creating a small amount of expectation to possibly hearing the worst news of their existence.

Usually, based on your demeanor and tone, family and loved ones know the news is coming. It is your job to be supportive by expressing your sincere condolences and sitting with them as long as you can. As a trainee, you can probably spend at least ten to fifteen minutes with them, or until you feel it is right to step away and let a family grieve in private.

A final reminder about your own mental health. Immediately after losing a patient, for you to continue to function as a provider, stay aware of the impact that the loss has had on you. Take a break if you need one—this seems like obvious advice, but not enough of us actually do it. Be certain that you are ready to give one hundred percent to the next patient, because however unfair it may seem given what you just experienced, your next patient's expectations never diminish.

HANDLING THE AFTERMATH

Patients who pass under your care may pose some of the most difficult situations that you will deal with, both inside and outside of work. Everyone has their kryptonite in terms of what kinds of cases will be especially emotional. For me, watching a parent witness their son or daughter's death continues to be one of the most devastating things to witness. As a senior resident, I will never forget the screaming mother running into our emergency department with a lifeless one-month-old boy, apneic, pulseless, and with hemoptysis.

While these experiences are often depressing and unforgettable, they also hold immense potential as learning opportunities. Learn from them by gathering your team members for a debriefing meeting. After a patient's death, debriefs should involve *every staff member even slightly involved in the case,* whether or not they are medical personnel. Even the clerk who had a brief interaction with the patient or their family should be involved.

Everyone involved needs to be invited to a debrief not only for their own mental well-being and to process the situation, but also because they provide an additional perspective to the scenario that is *invaluable*, whether or not you immediately appreciate it.

A debrief can take many forms. In emergency medicine, as in most specialties, the code leader usually offers a debrief session during the same shift in which the patient passed. Typically, this provider will summarize the case, thank everyone for their hard work, comment on the strengths of team efforts, and obtain feedback on what could have been improved.

It is not unreasonable to have any staff member begin the discussion, as long as everyone has a chance to speak.

Sometimes the moment is too emotionally charged for staff to begin a debrief. In these cases, delay the debrief or hold a second one when all parties are ready to contribute their perspective.

16

Assessing Capacity

Imagine a patient who causes themselves harm after they left the hospital against your advice. Not only will you find yourself burdened by guilt, you might be litigated for not having deemed them to lack *compos mentis* (their sanity). Of course, not all patients who leave against your advice lack their sanity, but it only takes one to slip through the cracks for you to be found liable, putting your license in jeopardy. Fortunately, litigation in this arena is rare.

A more common problem as it pertains to assessing decision-making capacity is that it can be an extreme time suck. If you don't have a system for doing it, you will go in circles, wasting unnecessary time going in and out of a patient's room, wavering on whether or not they are "allowed" to refuse this treatment or that.

Finally, the reason you should give early thought to assessing capacity is that it arises as one of the most complex aspects of residency practice.[68] Consider an elderly person with early- or middle-stage dementia, with some superimposed delirium from a toxic-metabolic process, like a UTI. The patient can seemingly parrot what you are telling them, but they lack insight into their illness, meaning they don't really understand how their disease process is affecting them.[69]

To determine a patient's capacity for making decisions on their own, focus on a patient's **insight** into their illness.[70] This is the most important way to analyze their lucidity. The caveat is **the more gravity the decision carries, the more insight you must require the patient to express.**

For example, if a patient wants to leave the hospital in (life-threatening) acute persistent ventricular tachycardia that is symptomatic, they had better convince you that they *fully* understand that death is likely, and sooner rather than later. Conversely, if a patient is making the decision to refuse a topical diphenhydramine you recommended for a pruritic mosquito bite, *little* insight is needed.

For a patient who needs IV antibiotics for cellulitis, but who also wants to leave the hospital against medical advice, more insight needs to be expressed than for that bug bite. Exactly how much insight is really up to the provider.

The way you assess insight is by listening to the patient recapitulate their diagnosis, treatment options, and related risks.[71] Have them put these items into their own words. Many patients with advanced dementia can repeat parts of a sentence you verbalize, but few will be able to reword or summarize succinctly. If a patient can give you a reworded version of what you said that contains *the meaning* of what you communicated, then they have some insight.

If a patient can give the *reasoning* as to why they are making a potentially risky choice, this consolidates the sense that they have adequate insight. If a patient tells you, "Look, I've lived long enough. I'm ninety-eight, and I've been to the hospital every week for the last year. I know that there is a good likelihood of my passing in the next few days without being admitted, but I choose to go home instead." There is no way you can take away their freedom to make this choice, regardless of whether you agree or disagree on moral grounds.

Technically, asking a patient to demonstrate the *reasoning* for their decision is not a requirement for them to have decision-making capacity, but it is a useful activity, especially if you are unsure if they actually have that capacity.

Consider a patient with cellulitis whom you have been taking care of for several hours in the emergency department, with whom you have had several in-depth conversations about their medical history and life in general, to the extent that you get the sense they are completely with it, *compos mentis*. If this person opts to leave the hospital instead of staying for continued IV antibiotics against your advice, they aren't really obligated to tell you why they have made that choice. It is always reasonable to ask, especially when you are unsure about capacity, as you will see in the example below. But this particular patient that you have already determined is quite mentally "with it" may simply not want to share why he does not wish to stay hospitalized. Maybe he has an event to attend, maybe he wants to go to a different hospital, who knows?

Next, consider a mildly demented patient who concurrently has an acute process like a urinary tract infection. Sometimes all it takes in an elderly person is a UTI to cause significant delirium, diminishing their decision-making capacity on whether it's safe to leave the hospital, for example. When you ask this patient questions, he or she may be able to give simple responses. However, when you ask for their *reason* for wanting to leave, they will be unable to articulate it. One major difference between this patient and the former is that you had already determined that the former was "with it" enough when they refused your medical advice. However, with the confused elderly patient, if you have not heard them put together speech that is substantially coherent, you can't let them leave.

NON-COERCIVE STRATEGIES
TO AVOID AN AMA

When considering those who *can* give you a legitimate reason for wanting to leave the hospital, but by doing so you believe will cause them grave harm, there are still a few strategies you can use to convince them to follow your medical advice. Before you request the patient fill out the Against Medical Advice (AMA) form and watch them walk out of the hospital, first *take an inquisitive position*. Ask kindly for their reasoning for refusing your medical advice. Sometimes they won't be forthcoming, but other times, you will get an answer that has an implementable solution.

If a patient tells you they are leaving because of a craving to smoke, offer a nicotine patch or gum. If they are worried about alcohol, or other types of withdrawal if admitted, tell them that hospitals are capable of monitoring and treating withdrawal.

Some providers argue against this approach, that this promotes drug abuse. I counter with this question: would you rather have a dead druggie, or one that at least has a chance to fight an infection by being hospitalized, and then go out into the world to try and stay sober? I also argue that it is better to foster a positive relationship with drug abusers, and let them know that you will treat their withdrawal. Do this to create a therapeutic alliance that might make them more likely to seek help from medical institutions in the future.

Don't forget that when inquiring about patients' reasoning for refusing care there is a tendency for providers to be upset that a patient is not taking our advice.[72] Sometimes physicians and patients suddenly clash, and the relationship turns south quickly, because the provider is offended the patient isn't doing "as they are told." Such emotionally charged behavior from the physician is not the best approach. Rather, be mindful that the patient is having a difficult day (or maybe an entire life), and that kindness and inquisitiveness is more likely to align them with your decisions than hostility or frustration.

Second, try calling the patient's primary care provider or specialists who know them well, because these providers may have strategies that have worked in the past to convince them to adhere to medical advice. At the very least, contacting the patient's provider coordinates follow-up.

Third, with the patient's permission, you can call a family member or friend. The patient may have wanted a loved one's input anyway. Consider calling them on speakerphone (again, with the patient's permission), so that all of your discussions are transparent. This can be very influential when trying to convince a patient to stay. "See, your brother agrees with me," or "I spoke with Dr. Levin, who knows you better than I do, and he supports the plan we have to admit you to the hospital." You will be surprised how quickly patients will respond when your plan suddenly includes an ally they are familiar with.

17

Self-care

As basic as it may sound, regular exercise, a well-thought-out on-shift meal plan, and a strategic sleep schedule will greatly improve your chances of success in training.

With adequate nutrition, you will be significantly sharper on-shift. Conversely, once you experience a long and challenging shift low on dietary fuel, you might become forgetful, or short with patients. For these reasons, do whatever it takes to ensure adequate on-shift meals through meal preparation, investing in a cooler, or incorporating meal supplements or shakes. Consider setting a timer to remind you to eat on busy days.

As discussed earlier, the importance of treating sleep as a sacred block of time is critical to success in training.[73] Some strategies that helped me get adequate sleep throughout residency included regular strenuous exercise, sleep hygiene tactics like avoiding late-night screen time and physically separating my bedroom from my work space, purchasing gear like ear plugs and a sleep mask or blackout shades, and utilizing a white noise app.

18

Innovation

In this brief section, I won't tell you the strategies that you should adopt to foster innovation, but I will emphasize that your training offers unprecedented opportunities to observe problems in healthcare that you can solve.

From the beginning of training, whether it is residency, PA, medical or nursing school, *pay attention* and keep notes documenting especially challenging problems and potential solutions. If nothing else, your notes can form a time capsule you can look back on and laugh at. But these notes may also be used for more, like developing a product or piece of literature.

Constantly ask yourself throughout training as many questions as you can to help understand why certain problems haven't been solved. Answer them to the best of your ability through research. Never let one, two, or a dozen naysayers prevent your progress.

Toward the end of residency, I noticed that the inclusion of residents in telehealth was lacking, but that the field held immense potential for resident involvement. At the same time, I calculated my hourly pay to be around $20 as a senior resident. I reflected on procedures I performed that week, from chest tubes to intubations, and realized that my wage did not match the relative challenge of these tasks. I then thought maybe there is a way to have residents perform simpler tasks through telehealth while improving their salary. In June 2018, I created the nation's first resident-run telemedicine company, Rezolve Telemed.

19

Conclusion

Residency can be an extremely challenging experience, especially because medical school curricula don't sufficiently prepare us for navigating the non-medical aspects of practice, including, but not limited to, team-building (or navigating inter-professional relationships), supporting colleague burnout, fostering excellence in bedside manner, optimizing patient perceptions of care, assessing patient decision-making capacity, discussing goals of care questions with patients, sharing prognoses with critically ill and employing end-of-life care strategies that maintain dignity and optimize comfort.

The so-called "hidden curriculum" can be taught, and this short text will hopefully begin a movement to do so early on at training institutions. The residency experience can be immensely more enjoyable for trainees and patients with this added guidance.

About the Author

Christopher Lee Taicher was born in Santa Monica, California. He trained on the East Coast for medical school (University of Vermont College of Medicine), internal medicine (Montefiore / Albert Einstein College of Medicine), and emergency medicine residency (Harvard / Massachusetts General Hospital and Brigham and Women's Hospital) before returning home to Los Angeles in 2019 to work as an attending emergency physician at Cedars Sinai Medical Center. Dr. Taicher is the founder and chief medical officer at Rezolve Telemed, the first telemedicine company comprised of a network of senior residents and fellows. His main interest is healthcare innovation. Dr Taicher's current attending position is held in Inglewood, California, in the Department of Emergency Medicine at Centinela Hospital Medical Center. Contact Chris at:

outofthestoneage@gmail.com

Notes

[1]Park, A. (2011, July 12). The July Effect: Why Summer Is The Most Dangerous Time To Go To The Hospital. *TIME.com*. Retrieved May 9, 2020, from https://healthland.time.com/2011/07/12/the-july-effect-why-summer-is-the-most-danger-ous-time-to-go-to-the-hospital/

[2]Medscape. (2019). *National physician burnout, depression & suicide report 2019.*

[3]Medscape. (2019). *National physician burnout, depression & suicide report 2019.*

[4]Vanderbilt, A. (1978). *The Amy Vanderbilt complete book of etiquette.* Garden City, NY: Doubleday Books.

[5]Tracy, B. (2002). *Eat that frog.* GABAL Verlag GmbH.

[6]Salles, A., Cohen, G. L., & Mueller, C. M. (2014). The relationship between grit and resident well-being. *The American Journal of Surgery, 207*(2), 251-254.; Zis, P., Anagnostopoulos, F., & Artemiadis, A. K. (2016). Residency training: Work engagement during neurology training. *Neurology, 87*(5), e45–e48.; Girard, D. E., & Hickam, D. H. (1991). Predictors of clinical performance among internal medicine residents. *J Gen Intern Med, 6*(2), 150–154.; Berger, L. (2019) Where does resiliency fit into the residency training experience: A framework for understanding the relationship between wellness, burnout, and resiliency during residency training. *Can Med Educ J 10*(1): e20–e27; Wortham, S. (2004). The interdependence of social identification and learning. *American Educational Research Journal, 41*(3), 715–750.

[7]ten Brinke, L., Vohs, K. D., & Carney, D. R. (2016). Can ordinary people detect deception after all? *Trends in Cognitive Sciences, 20*(8), 579-88.

[8]Spitzberg, B. H. (n.d.). (Re)Introducing communication competence to the health professions. *J Public Health Res, 2*(3), 23.; Friend, T.H., Jennings, S.J., Copenhaver, M.S. et al. (2017). Implementation of the Vocera Communication System in a Quaternary Perioperative Environment. *J Med*

Syst, 41(6). https://doi.org/10.1007/s10916-016-0652-9; Mathew, R., Weil, A., Sleeman, K. E., Bristowe, K., Shukla, P., Schiff, R., Flanders, L., Leonard, P., Minton, O., & Wakefield, D. (2019). The Second Conversation project: Improving training in end of life care communication among junior doctors. *Future Healthcare J*, 6(2), 129-136; Gordon, J.E., Deland, E., & Kelly, R. (2015) Let's talk about improving communication in healthcare. *Col Med Rev*, 1(1):23-27. doi: 10.7916/D8RF5T5D.

[9]Stanford Graduate School of Business. (2014, December 4). *Think fast, talk smart: Communication techniques* [Video]. YouTube. https://youtu.be/HAnw168huqA.

[10]Voss, Chris. Teaching the Art of Negotiation, Master Class. Video lecture.

[11]Fisher, R., & Ury, W. (2011). *Getting to Yes: Negotiating agreement without giving in*. Penguin Books.

[12]Komase, Y., Watanabe, K., Imamura, K., & Kawakami, N. (2019). Effects of a newly developed gratitude intervention program on work engagement among Japanese workers. *Journal of Occupational and Environmental*

Medicine, (61)9, e378-e383.doi: 10.1097/ JOM.0000000000001661 Kini, P., Wong, J., McInnis, S., Gabana, N., & Brown, J. W. (2016). The effects of gratitude expression on neural activity. *NeuroImage*, *128*, 1-10.

[13]Ajaz, A., David, R., Brown, D., Smuk, M., & Korszun, A. (2016). BASH: Badmouthing, attitudes and stigmatisation in healthcare as experienced by medical students. *BJPsych Bull*, *40*(2), 97-102; Ortiz-León S, Jaimes-Medrano AL, Tafoya-Ramos SA, Mujica-Amaya ML, Olmedo-Canchola VH, Carrasco-Rojas JA (2014) Experiences of bullying in medical residents. *Cir Cir*, *82*(3):290-301; Karan, A. (2017) Medical students need to be quizzed, but 'pimping' isn't effective. *STAT*. https:// www.statnews.com/2017/02/03/medical-stu- dents-pimping-testing-knowledge/; Foster, K., Roche, M., Giandinoto, J., & Furness, T. (2020). Workplace stressors, psychological well being, resilience, and caring behaviours of mental health nurses: A descriptive correla- tional study. (2020) *Int J Mental Health Nurse*, *29*(1), 56-58.

[14]Abedini, N. C., Stack, S. W., Goodman, J. L., & Steinberg, K. P. (2018). "It's not just time off": A

framework for understanding factors promoting recovery from burnout among internal medicine residents. *Journal of Graduate Medical Education*, *10*(1), 26-32.

[15]Medscape. (2019). *National physician burnout, depression & suicide report 2019*.

[16]Beaver, L. (2018). The US telehealth market: The market, drivers, threats, and opportunities for incumbents and newcomers. *Business Insider Intelligence Report*.

[17]Lee Roze des Ordons, A., de Groot, J. M., Rosenal, T., Viceer, N., & Nixon, L. (2018). How clinicians integrate humanism in their clinical workplace—'Just trying to put myself in their human being shoes'. *Perspect Med Educ*, *7*(5), 318-324; Kahn, P. A. (2017). The dawn of quantified humanism. *Journal of Graduate Medical Education*, *9*(4), 549; Martimianakis, M. A., Michalec, B., Lam, J., Cartmill, C., Taylor, J. S., & Hafferty, F. W. (2015). Humanism, the hidden curriculum, and educational reform. *Academic Medicine*, *90*, S5-S13.

[18]Merel, S. E., McKinney, C. M., Ufkes, P., Kwan, A. C., & White, A. A. (2016). Sitting at patients' bedsides may improve patients' perceptions of

physician communication skills. *J. Hosp. Med.*, *11*(12), 865-68; Swayden, K. J., Anderson, K. K., Connelly, L. M., Moran, J. S., McMahon, J. K., & Arnold, P. M. (2012). Effect of sitting vs. standing on perception of provider time at bedside: A pilot study. *Patient Education and Counseling*, *86*(2), 166-71.

[19]Bailoor, K., Valley, T., Perumalswami, C., Shuman, A. G., DeVries, R., & Zahuranec, D. B. (2018). How acceptable is paternalism? A survey-based study of clinician and nonclinician opinions on paternalistic decision making. *AJOB Empirical Bioethics*, *9*(2), 91-98.

[20]Schaffer, A. C., Jena, A. B., Seabury, S. A., Singh, H., Chalasani, V., & Kachalia, A. (2017). Rates and characteristics of paid malpractice claims among US physicians by specialty, 1992-2014. *JAMA Intern Med*, *177*(5), 710.; Kornmehl, H., Singh, S., Adler, B. L., Wolf, A. E., Bochner, D. A., & Armstrong, A. W. (2018). Characteristics of medical liability claims against dermatologists from 1991 through 2015. *JAMA Dermatol*, *154*(2), 160.

[21]Edgoose JY, Regner CJ, Zakletskaia LI. (2014). Difficult patients: Exploring the patient

perspective. *Fam Med, 46*(5):335-9.; Teo AR, Du YB, Escobar JI. (2013). How can we better manage difficult patient encounters. *Fam Pract, 62*(8):414-21.

[22]Dahan, S., Ducard, D., & Caeymaex, L. (n.d.). Apology in cases of medical error disclosure: Thoughts based on a preliminary study. *PLoS ONE, 12*(7), e0181854; Dudzinski, DM., Alvarez, C. (2017). Repairing "difficult" patient-clinician relationships, AMA J Ethics, *19*(4), 364-368. doi: 10.1001/journalofethics.2017.19.4.medu3-1704.

[23]Goodenough Company. (n.d.) *Goodenough Company, Inc.* http://37.60.229.246/~joycebal/test1/

[24]Grissinger, M. (2010). Disrespectful behavior in health care: Its impact, why it arises and persists, and how to address it—part 2. *Medication Errors, 42*(2): 74-75, 77.

[25]Kollar, J. (2016). Communication within the health care team: Doctors and nurses. *Orv Hetil, 157*(17):659-63. doi: 10.1556/650.2016.30444.

[26]Forbes, T. H., Larson, K., Scott, E. S., & Garrison, H. G. (2020). Getting work done: A grounded theory study of resident physician value of nursing communication. *Journal*

of Interprofessional Care, 34(2), 225-232. doi: 10.1080/13561820.2019.1631764.

[27]Hunt, E. A., Jeffers, J., McNamara, L., Newton, H., Ford, K., Bernier, M., Tucker, E. W., Jones, K., O'Brien, C., & Dodge, P. (2018). Improved cardiopulmonary resuscitation performance with CODE ACES 2: A resuscitation quality bundle. *JAHA, 7*(24).

[28]Spencer, S. A., Nolan, J. P., Osborn, M., & Georgiou, A. (2019). The presence of psychological trauma symptoms in resuscitation providers and an exploration of debriefing practices. *Resuscitation,* 142:175-181. doi: 10.1016/j.resuscitation.2019.06.280.; Coppens, I., Verhaeghe, S., Van Hecke, A., & Beeckman, D. (2018). The effectiveness of crisis resource management and team debriefing in resuscitation education of nursing students: A randomized controlled trial. *J Clin Nurs, 27*(1-2), 77-85.

[29]Hendrix, J. (2013). *Starting at zero.* Heyne Verlag.

[30]About: Aspire for Equality (2018). https://www.aspireforequality.com/about/

[31]Houpy, J. C., Lee, W. W., Woodruff, J. N., & Pincavage, A. T. (2017). Medical student

resilience and stressful clinical events during clinical training. *Medical Education Online*, *22*(1), 1320187; Arruda, W. (2015). Why failure is essential to success. *Forbes*. https://www.forbes.com/sites/williamarruda/2015/05/14/why-failure-is-essential-to-success/#33e8ea97923f

[32]Thorndike, T.D.S., Monteiro, J.F., McGarry, K. (2013). Mindfulness in residency: A survey of residents' perceptions on the utility and efficacy of mindfulness meditation as a stress-reduction tool. *R I Med J, 102*(3):29-33.; Sutton, A. (2019). Measuring the effects of self-awareness: Construction of the Self-Awareness Outcomes Questionnaire. *Eur. J. Psychol.*, *12*(4), 645–658.

[33]Damasio, A. (2008). *Descartes' error*. Random House.

[34]Considine, J., Botti, M., & Thomas, S. (2007). Do knowledge and experience have specific roles in triage decision-making? *Acad Emergency Med, 14*(8), 722–726.; Choi, Y. F. (2006). Triage rapid initial assessment by doctor (TRIAD) improves waiting time and processing time of the emergency department. *Emergency Medicine Journal*, *23*(4), 262-265; Bate, L., Hutchinson, A., Underhill, J., & Maskrey, N. (2012a). How clinical decisions

are made. *Br J Clin Pharmacol, 74*(4), 614–620. doi: 10.1111/j.1365-2125.2012.04366.x.

[35]Damasio, A. (2008). *Descartes' Error: Emotion, Reason, and the Human Brain*. Random House.

[36]Boushra, M. (2019). A second to get over it. *Annals of Emergency Medicine, 73*(5), 543–544.

[37]Sharp, B. R., Brownson, M., Thompson, R., Golden, S. K., Patterson, B., Pothof, J., Lee, A., et al. (2014). 280 pardon the interruption(s): Enabling a safer emergency department sign-out. *Annals of Emergency Medicine, 64*(4), S99.

[38]Helms, A. S., Perez, T. E., Baltz, J., Donowitz, G., Hoke, G., Bass, E. J., & Plews-Ogan, M. L. (2012a). Use of an appreciative inquiry approach to improve resident sign-out in an era of multiple shift changes. *J GEN INTERN MED, 27*(3), 287–291. 4

[39]Duijn, C. C. M. A., Welink, L. S., Bok, H. G. J., & ten Cate, O. T. J. (2018). When to trust our learners? Clinical teachers' perceptions of decision variables in the entrustment process. *Perspect Med Educ, 7*(3), 192–199.

[40]Wittich, C. M., Burkle, C. M., & Lanier, W. L. (2014). Medication errors: An overview

for clinicians. *Mayo Clinic Proceedings, 89*(8), 1116–1125. 7

[41]Dahan, S., Ducard, D., & Caeymaex, L. (n.d.). Apology in cases of medical error disclosure: Thoughts based on a preliminary study. *PLoS ONE, 12*(7), e0181854.

[42]Sherman, J. M., Chang, T. P., Ziv, N., & Nager, A. L. (2020). Barriers to effective teamwork relating to pediatric resuscitations. *Pediatric Emergency Care*, 36 (3), e146-e150. doi: 10.1097/PEC.0000000000001275.

[43]Bourdage, J. S., Wiltshire, J., & Lee, K. (n.d.). Personality and workplace impression management: Correlates and implications. *Journal of Applied Psychology, 100*(2), 537–546.

[44]Shappell, E. (Ed.) (2018). *MD in the Black: A Personal Finance Primer for Medical Residents.* USA: MD Fundamentals.

[45]Tabatabaee, A., Tafreshi, M., Rassouli, M., Aledavood, S., AlaviMajd, H., & Farahmand, S.K. (2016). Effect of therapeutic touch on pain related parameters in patients with cancer: A randomized clinical trial. *Mater Sociomed, 28*(3), 220.

[46]Kerr, F., Wiechula, R., Feo, R., Schultz, T., & Kitson, A. (2019). Neurophysiology of human touch and eye gaze in therapeutic relationships and healing. *JBI Database of Systematic Reviews and Implementation Reports, 17*(2), 209–247.

[47]Ma, J., Lee, D. K. K., Perkins, M. E., Pisani, M. A., & Pinker, E. (2019). Using the shapes of clinical data trajectories to predict mortality in ICUs. *Critical Care Explorations, 1*(4), e0010.

[48]Dubovsky, S. L., Antonius, D., Ellis, D. G., Ceusters, W., Sugarman, R. C., Roberts, R., Kandifer, S., et al. (2017). A preliminary study of a novel emergency department nursing triage simulation for research applications. *BMC Res Notes, 10*(1).

[49]Choi, Y. F. (2006). Triage rapid initial assessment by doctor (TRIAD) improves waiting time and processing time of the emergency department. *Emergency Medicine Journal, 23*(4), 262–265. 4

[50]Freeman, S., Eddy, S.L., McDonough, M., Smith, M.K., Okoroafor, N., Jordt, H., & Wenderoth, M.P. (2014). Active learning increases student performance in science, engineering, and mathematics. *Proc Natl Acad Sci USA, 111*: 8410–8415.

[51]Noorbakhsh-Sabet, N., Zand, R., Zhang, Y., & Abedi, V. (2019). Artificial intelligence transforms the future of health care. *The American Journal of Medicine, 132*(7), 795-801.

[52]Chen, Y., Elenee Argentinis, J., & Weber, G. (2016). IBM Watson: How cognitive computing can be applied to big data challenges in life sciences research. *Clinical Therapeutics, 38*(4), 688-701.

[53]Gabayan, G. Z., Gould, M. K., Weiss, R. E., Derose, S. F., Chiu, V. Y., & Sarkisian, C. A. (2017). Emergency department vital signs and outcomes after discharge. *Acad Emerg Med, 24*(7), 846-854.

[54]Cook, D. A., Pencille, L. J., Dupras, D. M., Linderbaum, J. A., Pankratz, V. S., & Wilkinson, J. M. (n.d.). Practice variation and practice guidelines: Attitudes of generalist and specialist physicians, nurse practitioners, and physician assistants. *PLoS ONE, 13*(1), e0191943.

[55]Joint Commission. (2009). *The Joint Commission guide to improving staff communication, 2nd ed.* Oakbrook Terrace, Illinois: Joint Commission Resources.; Brigham and Women's Hospital Department of Medicine. (n.d.) *Standards for physician communication.*; Kripalani, S., LeFevre, F., Phillips, C.O., Williams, M.V., Basaviah, P., & Baker, D.W.

(2007). Deficits in communication and information transfer between hospital-based and primary care physicians: Implications for patient safety and continuity of care. *JAMA, 297*(8): 831-41.

[56]Wang, J. K., Ouyang, D., Hom, J., Chi, J., & Chen, J. H. (n.d.). Characterizing electronic health record usage patterns of inpatient medicine residents using event log data. *PLoS ONE, 14*(2), e0205379.

[57]https://www.abms.org/board-certification/a-trusted-credential/based-on-core-competencies/

[58]Walker, M. (2017). *Why we sleep.* Penguin UK.

[59]EHRIntelligence. (2018). What are the benefits of clinical documentation improvement (CDI)? *EHRIntelligence.*

[60]EHRIntelligence. (2018). What are the benefits of clinical documentation improvement (CDI)? *EHRIntelligence.*

[61]Milano, A., Stankewicz, H., Stoltzfus, J., & Salen, P. (n.d.). The impact of a standardized checklist on transition of care during emergency department resident physician change of shift. *WestJEM, 20*(1), 29-34.

[62]Wittich, C. M., Burkle, C. M., & Lanier, W. L. (2014). Medication errors: An overview for clinicians. *Mayo Clinic Proceedings, 89*(8), 1116–1125.

[63]Lawrence, D. S., Masood, N., Astles, D., Fitzgerald, C. E., & Bari, A. Ul. (2015). Impact of pharmacist-led medication reconciliation on admission using electronic medical records on accuracy of discharge prescriptions. *J Pharm Pract Res, 45*(2), 166–173.; Leape, L. L. (1999). Pharmacist participation on physician rounds and adverse drug events in the intensive care unit. *JAMA, 282*(3), 267.

[64]McEvoy, J. W., Shatzer, J. H., Desai, S. V., & Wright, S. M. (2019). Questioning style and pimping in clinical Education: A quantitative score derived from a survey of internal medicine teaching faculty. *Teaching and Learning in Medicine, 31*(1), 53–64.

[65]Bandura, A. (1994). Self-efficacy. In V. S. Ramachaudran, ed., *Encyclopedia of Human Behavior* (Vol. 4, pp. 71-81). New York: Academic Press. (Reprinted in H. Friedman [Ed.] (1998). *Encyclopedia of Mental Health*. San Diego: Academic Press).

[66]Rattray, N.A., Ebright, P., Flanagan, M.E. et al. (2018). Content counts, but context makes the difference in developing expertise: A qualitative study of how residents learn end of shift handoffs. *BMC Med Educ* 18, 249.

[67]Clark, P. (2007). Medical futility: Legal and ethical analysis. *Journal Of Ethics | American Medical Association, 9*(5), 375-83. doi: 10.1001/virtualmentor.2007.9.5.msoc1-0705.

[68]Courtwright, A. M., Abrams, J., & Robinson, E. M. (2017). The role of a hospital ethics consultation service in decision-making for unrepresented patients. *Bioethical Inquiry, 14*(2), 241-250.

[69]Spooner, K. K., Salemi, J. L., Salihu, H. M., & Zoorob, R. J. (2017). Discharge against medical advice in the United States, 2002-2011. *Mayo Clinic Proceedings, 92*(4), 525-535.

[70]Ellajosyula, R., & Hegde, S. (2016). Capacity issues and decision-making in dementia. *Ann Indian Acad Neurol, 19*(5), 34.

[71]Owen, G. S., David, A. S., Richardson, G., Szmukler, G., Hayward, P., & Hotopf, M. (2009). Mental capacity, diagnosis and insight in psychiatric

in-patients: a cross-sectional study. *Psychol. Med.,*
39(8), 1389–1398.

[72]David, A.S. (1990) Insight and psychosis. *The British*
Journal of Psychiatry, 156: 798-808; Amador,
X.F., Strauss, D.H., Yale, S.A., Flaum, M.M.,
Endicott, J., Gorman, J.M. (1993) Assessment of
insight in psychosis. *American Journal of Psychiatry,*
150(6): 873-9.

[73]Heszen-Klemens, I. (1987). Patients' noncompliance
and how doctors manage this. *Social Science &*
Medicine, 24(5), 409–416.